THE BATTLES TO SAVE THE NHS

Universal, Free and Comprehensive

Piyush Pushkar

BRISTOL
UNIVERSITY
PRESS

First published in Great Britain in 2026 by

Bristol University Press
University of Bristol
1–9 Old Park Hill
Bristol
BS2 8BB
UK
t: +44 (0)117 374 6645
e: bup-info@bristol.ac.uk

Details of international sales and distribution partners are available at bristoluniversitypress.co.uk

DOI: 10.51952/9781529246094

British Library Cataloguing in Publication Data
A catalogue record for this book is available from the British Library

ISBN 978-1-5292-4607-0 paperback
ISBN 978-1-5292-4608-7 ePub
ISBN 978-1-5292-4609-4 OA Pdf

Cover design: Liam Roberts Design
Front cover image: Stocksy/Valeriya Simantovskaya
Bristol University Press uses environmentally responsible print partners.
Printed and bound in Great Britain by CPI Group (UK) Ltd, Croydon, CR0 4YY

Bristol University Press' authorised representative in the European Union is:
Easy Access System Europe, Mustamäe tee 50, 10621 Tallinn, Estonia,
Email: gpsr.requests@easproject.com

FSC
www.fsc.org
MIX
Paper | Supporting responsible forestry
FSC® C013604

Acknowledgements

I will always be grateful to all the activists, managers and politicians who gave me their time and confidence. Some of you also provided comments on drafts of chapters. The time and dedication you show to the cause never fails to amaze me. And a huge, special thanks to Emma Runswick for going on the record and being honest enough to disagree with me where you thought I was wrong or missing something.

My first forays into anthropological research were guided by Karen Sykes and Adam Brisley. I can't imagine what life would have been like without those three-hour discussions about William Blake, E.P. Thompson and Claude Lévi-Strauss. (And the goss about the 'moral' anthropologists.) Ruth Prince and Katie Smith, you were both wonderfully supportive and stimulating viva examiners, and I have benefited from your ongoing support. César Abadía-Barrero, your academic work always inspired me even before we met.

Laurence Cox, thank you for your support with the first version of the proposal for this book. And thanks for the idea of swapping round Chapters 1 and 2. Laura Portwood-Spacer, you didn't directly influence this book, but your *Book Proposal Book* certainly helped me write my proposal.

At Bristol University Press, Emily Ross and Anna Richardson, thank you for your unwavering support.

I must thank all the people supporting my current research. If I didn't have my current post, I wouldn't have had time to write this book. So thank you to Jenny Shaw, Andrew Irving, Andrew Shepherd, Louise Robinson and Tom Hewson. And, of course, everyone who has supported me in my clinical work: Hany El-Metaal, Caroline Cooper, Rukyya Hassan, Su Farrell, Simon Plunkett, John Crosby, Panchu Xavier, Lucy Bacon, Clare Oakley, not to mention my fellow specialist trainees and, of course, all the nurses, psychologists, administrators, domestic staff, support workers and others.

My loved ones, I won't name you. I couldn't have done this, or indeed anything, without you.

Contents

The research on which this book is based was funded by a Wellcome Trust fellowship [203337/Z/16/Z].

Chapter 4 is largely based on a previously published paper: Pushkar, Piyush. 2023. "Accountabilities in the NHS: Coercion, Finance and Responsibility." *The Cambridge Journal of Anthropology* 41 (1): 118–136. https://doi.org/https://doi.org/10.3167/cja.2023.410109.

Introduction

> Save the NHS.
> Save the NHS.
> *A chant commonly heard at NHS protests*

Shortly after starting the ethnographic fieldwork that this book is based on, my wife's waters broke. We picked up our bags, laid down an absorbent pad in the car, and went to hospital a jumble of nerves and emotions. Fear and anxiety regarding what might happen next and how that might affect us. *Not* fear regarding whether or how we could access maternity care, nor fear of how much it might cost us; we have never had to pay for healthcare.

About a year later, our son was admitted to hospital with an infection. We stayed in hospital a few days while he was treated with intravenous antibiotics. On the day that we were discharged, we put our son in a vest that said 'BORN IN THE NHS'. The doctors and nurses loved it. The written message touched them in some way. He was not just born and cared for in this hospital, by these doctors, nurses and midwives. He was born *in the NHS*. The doctors, nurses and midwives worked *in the NHS*. The *NHS* meant something to us, and it meant something to them.

The NHS is England's public healthcare system.[1] But if that is all it is, why have I spent the past few years – pretty much a decade – trying to figure out what it is? What *is* the NHS? What do people imagine that it is? And how does that relate to ideas of what it was, what it could be, and what it ought to be? An institution that delivers healthcare? A decaying remnant of the UK's welfare state? A 'national religion', as one former Conservative[2] MP once described it?

This book traces a battle over what the NHS is, how people remember its history, what it means, and what it symbolizes. My argument is based not just on the stories activists, clinicians, bureaucrats and politicians told me about what the NHS *does*, but also on their moral imagination: of the NHS, of the state, of society and of socialism. I spent 13 months with political activists campaigning to 'save the NHS' (hereafter NHS activists). I asked why they felt it needed saving and why they felt it *ought* to be saved. But also, what was it that they felt they were protecting?

They were protesting governmental policy. But as anthropologists Cris Shore and Susan Wright (2011) note, policies are always contested. By looking at how and why people disagree, we can better understand the relationships and power dynamics that shape how the policies are created, effected and interpreted, but also how they are mobilized within various moral projects. My primary focus will be on activists, among whom there were often differences of opinion. But the key 'interpretive battles' (Ginsburg, 1989: 96) were between activists and state actors[3] – managers and politicians – advocating reforms. I will describe how the imagination of the NHS crystallized in the moral arguments that activists used in political confrontation. What values coalesced around activists' struggles in these 'policy worlds' (Shore and Wright, 2011: 8), with what consequences for whom?

In the moral economy shaped and sustained by the enactment of fiscal austerity and public service reforms in the face of widespread opposition and abundant evidence of the harm caused by that austerity, NHS activists understood the NHS as a symbol of the good society, a society whose members undertook to take collective responsibility for one another. They understood the NHS, the Labour Party and UK society in general as having changed for the worse to accommodate neoliberalism over the previous decades, with a sharp recent deterioration as a result of austerity. However, they still maintained a conceptualization of the NHS as being directly opposed to the individual responsibilization (Rose, 2000) they associated with neoliberalism, and to Margaret Thatcher's dictum that 'There is no such thing as society'. NHS activists believed that we *do* live in a society, and that the NHS represented the basic elements of how members of a society should treat one another. More specifically, they understood the NHS as an example of how the state can and should play a role in contributing to the realization of the good society. The changes that they feared in the NHS represented a potential failure of the state to uphold its obligations to the people of England.

Most of the NHS activists with whom I worked understood themselves as socialists, they understood socialism as pertaining to finding ways to live together in solidarity and mutual responsibility, rather than competition, and they understood the NHS as an example of actually existing socialism. That is, it was a symbol, but not *just* a symbol. It was a real structure existing in the UK state, that they had particular memories of, which they could mobilize in the construction of moral arguments to take into political conflicts. Since the NHS already existed, NHS activists interpreted cuts and privatization as threats to the enactment of such solidarity and mutual responsibility.

The next two sections discuss the book's theoretical framework and methodology. Non-academic readers may wish to skip straight to Chapter 1.

Moral economy, group formation and class consciousness

This is a work of political anthropology that draws heavily on the anthropology of ethics. I integrate these two fields within a moral economy framework. E.P. Thompson (1991a) used the moral economy formulation to explain how eighteenth-century peasants and workers apprehended changes in how social relations between groups contributed to the ways in which goods – particularly food – were exchanged between them.[4] Changes in social relations had economic consequences, namely the price of bread became unaffordable. The people who then could not afford to eat understood these changes as morally wrong. They constructed their arguments for why it was wrong by drawing on how they remembered the past; they argued that the rich were foregoing their obligation to the poor by allowing bread to become unaffordable. Such an argument made an appeal to older alliances between social groups – between peasants and landowners – while also contributing to the formation of new solidarities on the basis of shared interests. People of various occupations realized that the new arrangement of economic relations made bread unaffordable for all of them, but that if they rioted together, they might force action from those in power.

Like Thompson's peasants, the activists I met contested changes to the structure of the NHS with moral arguments based on their own understandings of the past. My research took place at a particular historical and political conjuncture, in the UK ten years after the 2008 global financial crash. In 2010, the Tory party won a general election, after 13 years of Labour government. The Tories formed a coalition government with the Liberal Democrat party. The coalition went on to enact severe cuts on most public services, including the NHS. Very quickly, a host of protest groups emerged and flourished, including Occupy and UK Uncut,[5] as well as smaller groups working locally. Most of the time, such groups did not advocate radical change; they simply sought to stop or reverse austerity, or to implore international corporations to pay taxes. It has been commonplace to describe the limited goals of these protest groups as conservative (e.g. Graeber, 2013). The inspiration I take from Thompson is in focusing on how these actors were trying out various arguments and strategies, forming new ties, solidarities and cleavages between groups.

At the same time, in 2018, anthropology was locked in a strange state of affairs, in which anthropologists of ethics viewed explanations of social action that prioritized structural forces with suspicion. Meanwhile, political and economic anthropologists viewed the anthropology of ethics' focus on individual reflection with equal suspicion.[6] Thankfully, anthropological theory has emerged from this adversarial hiatus while still maintaining the productive diversity of differing theoretical understandings of morality.[7] For example, the recent *Cambridge Handbook for the Anthropology of Ethics*, edited by James Laidlaw, includes a chapter on *Activism and Political Organization*, in which Sian Lazar uses Argentine trade unions to argue that the resilience of labour activism under adverse economic and political conditions depends on 'projects of collective ethical-political self-construction' (Lazar, 2023: 792). That is, the political actions of the institution depend on the ethical reflections of its members.

In the Introduction (2023) of the same book, Laidlaw responds to critics of the anthropology of ethics. He agrees with Sherry Ortner that much of what she had labelled 'dark anthropology' (Ortner, 2016: 47; Laidlaw, 2023: 4) was theoretically arid, insofar as it sought to explain ethics and morality as local, epiphenomenal responses to globally applicable structural forces: power, oppression, exploitation, inequality. Laidlaw refers to such scholarship as 'the explaining away of what people understand to be their motivations, values, ideals, and aspirations as no more than the effects of postulated entities, structures, or forces, imagined as existing on a larger scale or at a deeper level or in a different temporal realm to the people whose conduct they are said to cause' (2023: 3). However, he acknowledges that not all contributors to the book share his theoretical viewpoint, that there is productive value in collegial diversity, and that part of the project of the anthropology of ethics is to infuse all of anthropology with a recognition that ethical evaluation is a part of all social life. He writes: 'Explicitly and implicitly, consistently and inconsistently, concertedly and by-the-way as they go about their everyday lives, [people] act in ways that constitute at least partial answers to the questions of how one ought to live and what kind of life is a good life' (2023: 1). They do so in social, cultural and institutional contexts, with political histories and present conditions that both constrain and structure the possibilities for those ethical evaluations.

I situate this book resolutely in the integrated camp, neither suspicious of treating ethical evaluations as social phenomena worthy of investigation, nor unwilling to incorporate discussions of economy or power into my analyses. Throughout the book I use theoretical tools from the anthropology of ethics, modified and retheorized for my field. However, it is only by applying these tools within a moral economy framework that I will be able to develop a holistic argument that understands the place of activists' moral[8] reasoning within political[9] battles over reforms of economic structures.

How can we make sense of the fact that the activists I did research with described themselves as socialists but often did not consider themselves Marxists? Largely retired professionals, they interpreted and mobilized the histories of socialism and Labour in ways that sometimes surprised me. They did not concentrate on the means of production, but instead talked about public ownership (by which they meant state ownership) and public provision of care for all; not just healthcare, but all forms of welfare. In their activism the NHS took precedence over other welfare institutions not because of the biopolitical importance of life and death, but because of the ongoing existence of the state institution that provided healthcare, even when other state welfare institutions had been lost, taken away by a malign elite in control of the state that was relinquishing its obligation to look after the public.

Thompson's disavowal of mechanical or 'vulgar materialist' explanations pushes us to focus on how workers themselves understood and voiced their experiences of exploitation and how this fed into how they *justified* their actions. The poor objected to the changes in the economy in *moral* terms:

> a consistent traditional view of social norms and obligations, of the proper economic functions of several parties within the community … taken together, can be said to constitute the moral economy of the poor. An outrage to these moral assumptions, quite as much as actual deprivation, was the usual occasion for direct action. ([1971] 1991a: 188)

Thompson restores to this group of oppressed people their agency through fine-grained analysis of the ways in which they *used* particular customs, inherited *and chosen* from the past, as tools in both apprehending and also protesting the present. Similarly, in his classic work, *The Making of the English Working Class* (1980), Thompson revolutionized the study of class, following a historiographical model that did not consider the material circumstances that people lived in as the simple, determining engine of social change. Instead, Thompson demonstrated how it was people's *experience* of those material circumstances, according to icons and understandings of self, identity and other – each with its own history – that contributed to whether people resisted, how they organized and how their mobilizations were understood by others. Human experience was the contingent mediator between base and superstructure.[10]

For Thompson, English peasant and worker mobilizations did not fit a pre-existing model of class; they developed their own class analysis. They united under broad, inclusive identifications, combining an ironic take on Burke's description of them as the 'swinish multitude' with Paine's rhetoric of (the) *Rights of Man*, along with a quasi-universal appeal to the 'freeborn Englishman'.[11] The usefulness of Thompson for this book arises from his emphasis on actors' *own* analyses and awareness of sides in the battles they fought, using their own icons and tropes. In our own political moment, in which actors are again forging their own putative class analyses to wield in battles – 'the 99%', 'the many not the few', 'precarious workers', 'white working class', 'liberal elites', 'No Kings' – I ask how activists' own class analyses (often but not always tacit) influence and are influenced by the values of the NHS – universal, free, comprehensive – as interpreted by activists. I found that conceptualizing a vision of socialism with the values of the NHS at its core had consequences for the kinds of alliances activists forged.

Thompson's concern with the contingency of historical progress gave him a view of culture not as a bounded site of consensus within a social group, but a site of conflict. He describes culture as being in continual flux (1991b), pointing not to shared understandings or 'webs of significance', but to disagreements and protests. The point is not that consensus did not exist, but that it had to be fought for, with a fragile and contingent consciousness built around this struggle. It is exactly such a solidaristic consciousness that I will trace, as it solidifies – albeit with some fragility – around the moral imagination of the NHS, *through* conflict with managers and politicians.

Thompson's protestors articulated their discontent by retelling and re-imagining past memories. Therefore, 'the moral economy is *summoned into being* in resistance to the economy of the "free market"… The rationalisations or "modernisations" of the capitalist market offended against community norms and *continually called into being* a "moral" antagonist' (Thompson, 1991b: 340, my emphasis). What moral economy and what moral antagonist was being summoned into being in the battles to save the NHS?

NHS activists drew a political battle line based on their moral imagination of the NHS. In so doing, they formed new social groups. Activists believed that the reforms they opposed would lead to privatization, and privatization was wrong. The state was foregoing an obligation to provide healthcare, to look after the people living in it. Activists considered that anyone advocating the current suite of reforms was the moral antagonist, or at least in coalition with the moral antagonist. On the other hand, activists themselves were protecting the NHS as a universal service for the whole population. Therefore, they implicitly considered themselves as in alliance with the whole population of the country, defined as expansively as possible. In activists' evaluations of how the NHS was changing now, their imagination of how the NHS ought to be combined with particular memories of how it once had been. In this process of apprehending the present, they did not just recall former social relations; they produced new potential social formations.

They narrated the history of the NHS in a particular way, choosing particular aspects of the past that allowed them to focus on particular values and state obligations that made particular kinds of coalitions between groups possible. I will elaborate on how activists focused on universality, defining it as broadly as possible, thus attempting to build alliances that spread beyond narrow interest groups or professions.

What is important, then, to an analysis of a developing consciousness, is a careful consideration of *which* aspects from *which past* fed into the imagination of the future. Furthermore, how did people use these memories to forge links and alliances with particular others; whom did they consider class compatriots and whom class enemies? How did moral arguments build on particular understandings of the past to undergird solidarity between workers of different backgrounds, and what limits did these understandings place on the imagination of the future?

Ethnographic method and positionality

I am a British doctor, working in the NHS. I completed medical school in Edinburgh in 2007, after which I moved to the Northwest of England, where I have remained since, except for six months working as an aeromedical retrieval doctor in Australia. I come from an affluent background; both of my parents are doctors who migrated from India to England just before I was born. My mother did not practise in the UK, but my father worked as a GP and rose up the ranks to become chair of the Clinical Commissioning Group in which he worked. He retired shortly after I finished fieldwork.

I was not politically active until the Tories came to power and began to enact fiscal austerity in state services. At that point, I began to attend anti-austerity protests and sign petitions. When the Health and Social Care Act (henceforth the Act) was announced in 2011, I became more involved in the campaigning side of political activism, joining groups including Keep our NHS Public and the Socialist Health Association, and writing blogs and articles. However, I remained on the fringes of these groups, only attending occasional meetings and not taking up any official positions. Since then, while continuing to work as a doctor in the NHS, I have remained engaged in campaigns against reforms.

In 2016, I became involved in an industrial dispute between junior doctors[12] and the government. Then Secretary of State for Health, Jeremy Hunt, had announced that he intended to impose a new contract for junior doctors. At the time, I was a union rep for the organization representing junior doctors, the British Medical Association. I helped organize pickets, I spoke to junior doctors and other staff within the hospital, I collected signatures from members of the public on petitions. I noticed that NHS activists and junior doctors appeared to form alliances during that campaign. I was one of the people doing the work of communicating with other unions, attending meetings of other activist groups, forging links with other people. I could see that it was in junior doctors' interest to gain the support of other groups, and that the industrial dispute was somehow connected to campaigns to save the NHS, but I had not yet formulated a coherent explanation of the relationship. I could see that NHS activists were waging a political battle using moral arguments: It was 'wrong' to close hospitals or reduce services. So we must 'save the NHS'. I was interested in why it was wrong to close hospitals, and how the leap was being made from a local struggle against a particular hospital closure, to a national struggle to 'save the NHS'. It appeared to me that the wrongness of NHS reconfigurations implied that activists sensed a rightness or a goodness about the NHS as it ought to be, but I struggled to pin it down. Therefore, I embarked on a PhD project to clarify what remained hazy for me. The fieldwork for that doctoral research involved 13 months of ethnographic fieldwork, mostly with activist groups campaigning to save, defend or protect the NHS from cuts and privatization.[13]

One of the groups that supported junior doctors in 2016 was Keep our NHS Public. I had been a member of the Greater Manchester branch of Keep our NHS Public (Greater Manchester KONP) for several years before starting fieldwork. The group were happy for me to attend groups more regularly, and to join in their other campaigning activities. At Greater Manchester KONP meetings, representatives from various affiliated campaigning organizations attended to give reports of local activities.

One of these groups was based in a part of Greater Manchester that I will call Dunning. I will call the group Dunning Keep Our NHS Public (henceforth Dunning KONP). I emailed the chair, Wes, who invited me to join them on one of their regular Tuesday morning protests, outside Dunning Hospital. After that, I became a regular attendee on Tuesday mornings, joined them for other protests in Dunning, as well as other parts of Manchester and London, attended their monthly organizing meetings, helped with stalls in Dunning town centre, and was grateful to be invited to their social gatherings, including the legendary annual Christmas party at Esther's house. I also conducted semi-structured interviews with nine of Dunning KONP's members, often in their homes or in local pubs.

At the protests, for two hours every week, we stood outside the hospital and chatted. We discussed music, television, climate change, fracking, Brexit, and the wider political scene in the UK. In other words, this was where I really got to know the members of Dunning KONP. When put together with the interviews and the organizing meetings, I began to understand how they perceived their role in influencing political decision-making in Dunning.

So protests and meetings were an integral part of my participant-observation.[14] Although meetings can be uniquely useful vantage points from which to study bureaucracy and social action (Abram, 2017; Brown, Reed and Yarrow, 2017), a full understanding of the social processes taking place in those meetings requires a lot of personal and contextual information that benefits from investigation outwith the meeting itself. Therefore, I interviewed as many activists as I could. In the second half of fieldwork, I organized lunches with groups of activists, where I fed back some early analyses to develop them in concert with activists. They helped me to make sense of my own fieldnotes and the things I had learned in previous interviews. Each interview was unique, an extraordinary encounter (Smith and Staples, 2015) that did not just provide material to be analysed, but was itself part of the ethnographic analysis. In total I interviewed 22 activists, some of them two or three times.

Members of Greater Manchester KONP, Dunning KONP and the Socialist Health Association often attended open meetings of the councils, the clinical commissioning groups (CCGs) or the hospital trusts. I attended these meetings with members of the groups, and occasionally attended alone as well. I also joined NHS activists when they organized private meetings with managers or politicians. I often heard managers and politicians speak at conferences or on TV, and read what they had said in newspapers. But most of my data with managers and politicians came from interviews.

I interviewed nine managers.[15] Of these nine, four were also clinicians.[16] These managers were mostly employed in senior positions of control at Clinical Commissioning Groups (CCGs), hospital trusts and the Greater Manchester Health and Social Care Partnership (GMHSCP).[17] I also interviewed 12 politicians, of whom 11 were local councillors[18] and one was a member of Parliament (MP).[19] MPs were not easy to gain access to. The one Labour MP that I did interview only had time for a 30-minute interview. None of the Conservative MPs replied to my emails. In contrast to the MPs, the councillors that I met were very easy to arrange interviews with.

Many activists were not concerned regarding anonymity. However, I have chosen to change everyone's names in the book, since not anonymizing some people would have compromised the anonymity of the other people who did want to remain anonymous. I have changed one place name as well: Dunning. I made this choice because tensions did run high at times between the various relevant organizations in Dunning, where some of my deepest ethnographic data comes from. As will become apparent in Chapter 5, what was at stake was not just trust and congeniality in relationships between people, but also people's jobs and livelihoods. I have also been deliberately vague with the exact positions held of some of the managers and politicians, as well as those activists who hold officer positions in activist organizations.[20]

Chapter overview

Chapter 1 – Children of the NHS

This chapter focuses on the life histories of two activists, Lily and Leroy, born in the 1940s and 1950s. Lily and Leroy remembered how the changes brought in by the Attlee government had helped them to lead happy and flourishing lives. They considered themselves socialists and they, like many of the activists I spoke to, thought of the NHS as a 'symbol of socialism'. But they were not anti-capitalist. Listening to what Lily and Leroy told me about the NHS and socialism helped me to understand exactly what the NHS meant to them, and where it drew its potency from. It was not just a collection of hospitals. And it was not just a symbol. It was an actually existing state structure, and thus an example of how the state could intervene in society to strengthen our collective responsibility to look after each other. The NHS showed that we care – and that the state could help us to care – for our fellow citizens.

The chapter engages the anthropology of ethics to theorize the significance of using a moral example/exemplar in this way. Namely, using their own interpretation of the NHS as an example draws it into an interpretive battle that places its moral meaning at the heart of political contestation.

Chapter 2 – Defending the Indefensible: How Did We Get Here?

This chapter describes the impossible situation that activists find themselves in. They are trying to save something that is not recognizable from their memory of what the NHS was. The chapter gives a short history of the NHS, according to the narrative as activists understood it. I furnish the narrative with historical detail and underline the importance of reckoning with the ways in which colonialism contributed to the foundations of the welfare state, a reckoning that was not lost on the activists I worked with. This colonial history provides context for interpretations of the NHS not just as icon of the state, but also of the nation, and even nationalism. But, ultimately, the key narrative that activists drew from their understanding of the history and present state of the NHS was that it was declining as a result of cuts and privatization, which therefore must be halted.

Chapter 3 – Fears of Privatization

Why are activists always predicting that the next suite of reforms is going to lead to privatization, to the end of the NHS? How has the future itself become something to be feared? This chapter takes the proposed creation of Accountable Care Organizations as a case example to examine why activists feared all reforms. NHS activists' fears of privatization drew on the empirical evidence gained from their own experiences, beginning with workplace struggles of trade union representatives in the 1990s, which provided ballast for the organizations that I spent time with. I situate their analyses within sociological critique of privatization, marketization and New Public Management. I interpret activists' fears as a potent critique of the vulnerability of the welfare state in the face of global capital. And yet, despite these threats from capital's attempts to undermine the state and parasitize state infrastructure, the NHS – and the fight to save it – continues to exist. Further, the NHS as activists imagined it stood out from other public services precisely because it represented the capacity of the state to stand up to the power of private capital in the name of the public good, as long as there were people willing to contribute to that struggle. However, I also identify a weakness in activists' critique. Where they focused their analytical attention depended on their moral understandings of what was to be protected: the existing structure of the NHS as a moral example. Therefore, they were caught out when the existing structure of general practice – rather than public service reforms proposed by contemporary state actors – provided a pathway for privatization.

Chapter 4 – Whose Side are NHS Managers on?

The NHS managers I spoke to expressed the same values as the activists, describing the NHS as 'universal, free and comprehensive'. So why were they in battle with these activists, often seeking to undercut or constrain their ethical vision? The difference between the two groups was that managers sought to realize their values within the financial constraints that were the precise point of contention for campaigners. Managers placed boundaries around what was achievable. Activists contested the political choice over where to place those boundaries. They brought morality into their political arguments, speaking about the consequences of cuts, thus re-exposing said choices to debate. Activists made the moral political by arguing that the reforms would result in a foregoing of the state's obligations to its citizens. Managers were immune to these moral arguments because – within the audit culture of an NHS directed under the auspices of New Public Management – their hands were tied. They were being forced to comply with centrally given directives. If they did not comply, they knew they would be sacked. They would be held accountable for fulfilling their perceived duty to balance the books. But when managers tried to narrow the space within which moral judgements could be made, they situated themselves in such a way that activists perceived them as in alliance with the 'moral antagonists' in the Tory Party.

Chapter 5 – NHS Activism, Socialism, and the Labour Party

This chapter traces the engagement between NHS activists and the Labour Party. I observe the similarities between activists' critique of the party and the New Left critique that emerged in the 1960s and developed through the 1970s. One key difference was that whereas the New Left sought to give a structural explanation for the 'betrayal' of the working classes and socialist goals by those in charge of the party, I saw such structural explanations become intertwined with individualized judgements of particular people. Therefore, activists strategized on the basis of a suspicion that a malign other was seeking to betray them, the Labour Party or their ethical vision of how the state or society should be remade. These suspicions were self-perpetuating and undermined potential alliances, fracturing solidarities rather than building coalitions. Focusing on more structural explanations may be more helpful for building solidarity.

Chapter 6 – NHS Workers and Industrial Power: An Interview with Emma Runswick

Since the end of my fieldwork there has been a change of ruling party in the UK. There have also been multiple industrial disputes across the public sector, including in the NHS. This chapter is a transcription of an interview that took place in April 2025, with Emma Runswick, deputy chair of British Medical Association council. We discuss health worker strikes and how they are related to activism against cuts and privatization in the NHS.

1

Children of the NHS

In 2011, I read about then Secretary of State for Health Andrew Lansley's plans for the Health and Social Care Bill.[1] He was trying to complete the marketization of the health service, a project started by Margaret Thatcher in the 1980s. I sensed something dangerous in what he was trying to do, something I should object to. So I gravitated towards campaigns to protect what we had, to 'save the NHS'. But from that very first day, I was haunted by a nagging question about the campaigns I found and joined: is NHS activism conservative? This might seem like an odd question to ask about these activists, of whom I am now one. These were people who often considered themselves to be socialists. But it is a criticism that is often thrown at NHS activists from opposing wings: either by managers and politicians attempting to push through reforms, or by radical left political commentators. The former claim that NHS activists are wedded to the status quo and simply resistant to *any* change. The latter are frustrated by activists' defensiveness; why 'save' or 'protect' the NHS? Why not expand and improve the NHS?[2]

In this first chapter, I tackle these questions by asking another question: what are NHS activists actually trying to save? What does the NHS mean to them? Once we have established what we are talking about when we talk about the NHS, only then can we move onto the strategies to defend it, to ask where those campaigns are leading, what consequences they are having, to see if they are conservative. So this chapter will do what anthropologists call 'thick description' (Geertz, 1973). I will not just describe what activists did and report what they said. I will interpret what their words and actions meant to them, within the sociopolitical and relational context in which they lived. Activists told me that the NHS was an example of 'actually existing socialism'. That, in a sense, is what the NHS meant to them. But saying this only begets further questions. The point of ethnographic research is not to illustrate settled meanings, but to map out the contours and consequences of battle. What did they mean by 'example'? More importantly, what did they mean by 'socialism'? The final section of the chapter will draw on the work of anthropologist Faye Ginsburg (1989) to show how this work of debating what words and concepts mean is itself a key battleground for political movements.

In the UK, progressive institutions and people who considered themselves on the left spent much of the 1990s and 2000s being discouraged from openly discussing socialism. New Labour took pains to suppress overt references to socialism. However, the period of quiet socialism is clearly over now. Keir Starmer's Labour Party may not be singing from the rooftops about economic planning or ownership of the means of production, but a socialist ecosystem has been revived, with new media organizations, podcasts, prominent media personalities, publishers, think tanks, reading groups, etc.[3] But we[4] are still finding our feet with how we discuss what socialism is, who socialists are, and what ends socialism ought to have in mind. The purpose of this chapter will be to look at what vision of society, and therefore what kind of socialism, was implicit in NHS activism. To do so, I will be using anthropological theories of how examples and exemplars work – what they do – in social life. So I begin with a brief description of how anthropologist Joel Robbins has theorized the moral example.

Robbins and the moral 'example'

According to Robbins, 'examples' (2015: 18) are 'representations that model the realization of single values in full form – forms that are not common in daily life because most actions are driven by a mix of diverse value considerations' (2015: 18). He follows the philosopher Alessandro Ferrara in arguing that the force of the example comes from having united the force of what *is* with the force of what *ought to be*. The example already is what ought to be. Not all actions could end up being examples of this nature, because most of the time life is too complicated. Even though all actions may be attempts to realize a value or several values, more often than not the existence in that social milieu of other values, other forces and other constraints will stop the initial value being fully realized.

Rituals are paradigmatic of what he means by examples, full realizations of some kind of value. Thus he argues that rituals are particularly useful to anthropologists interested in the values of societies being studied. To explicate his theory, he uses Papua New Guinean Urapmin rituals that are examples of the opposing values of individualism and relationality. To perform rituals, whether religious (e.g. baptism of an infant), political (e.g. coronation of a sovereign), educational (e.g. graduation of a student), or otherwise, people generally construct a specific, curated space, separated from the complications of daily life. It is this special space that is afforded for the ritual that allows the relevant value to be fully realized, free from the constraints that normally hinder them.

The fact that in the simplified space of the ritual the value was fully realized does not compel people to also attempt to fully realize those values in everyday life. Robbins states that this would be impossible because other values, other forces would get in the way, 'but their ritual accomplishment none the less remains in play in the rushed flux of everyday life; indeed, it remains in play in the form of people's possession of examples that will henceforth solicit some of their energy towards further realization of the value(s) involved' (2015: 22).

Let us keep Robbins' model in mind as I describe how NHS activists hold the NHS as a moral example, realizing a set of values. My use of the example will differ from Robbins in one key respect. Far from existing in a special space set back from daily life, the force of the NHS as an example stems exactly from the fact that it has existed, and continues to exist, without a special space carved out for it, even in the face of a neoliberal capitalist system. This chapter will argue that it is the NHS's existence as a moral example – rather than the biopolitical importance of healthcare over other state services – that begins to explain why the NHS matters more than other welfare organizations. The NHS demonstrated the capacity for the realization of certain values that seemed at odds with neoliberal capitalism. In the words of Erik Olin Wright (2013), it was a real utopia, its viability proven by its actual existence. When I asked the chair of Greater Manchester Keep our NHS Public (KONP), Leon, what was good about the NHS, he simply said 'It's *there*'.

But *what* is '*there*'? NHS activists are not campaigning for what there *is*. Activists are campaigning for what they imagine there *ought to be*, incorporating many elements of what there *used to be*. On the other hand, the NHS does exist *now*. And it is this fact that allows the full realization of NHS values to remain 'in play in the rushed flux of everyday life' (Robbins, 2015: 22). The imagined and the actual NHS remain in tension, but the very fact of the NHS's ongoing existence facilitates the ongoing possession in activists' minds of the imagined NHS as example, 'that will henceforth solicit some of their energy towards further realization of the value(s) involved' (Robbins, 2015: 22).

Children of the NHS

One of the first things I noticed at activist meetings and protests was the abundance of grey hair. In Dunning KONP, I was one of two people that attended the Tuesday morning protests that had not yet retired. The other protestors welcomed me with open arms, partly because of my youth. (I was born in the early 1980s. I do not consider myself young. But other activists often did.) Members of Dunning KONP often talked about this age discrepancy, joking that my presence brought down the average age by ten years.

The difference in age was important for how we understood the world, local politics and the place of the NHS. The other members of Dunning

KONP brought different memories, stories and narratives to their activism than the ones I brought to mine. Over the course of 13 months together, I got to learn about their personal histories, as well as the history of the NHS and the UK as they understood it. For them, three time periods stood out: the post-war period under Clement Attlee's Labour government; the 1980s under Margaret Thatcher's Conservative government; and the 2010s under David Cameron's coalition and then majority Conservative governments. Learning about how they remembered these periods helped me to understand what they felt was happening to the NHS, and why it was wrong. Referring to how close their own birthdates were to that of the NHS, some within a couple of years, they described themselves as 'children of the NHS'. They remembered Thatcher, they remembered the miners' strikes of the 1980s, they remembered free orange juice and cod liver oil, provided by the NHS. Moreover, they remembered the things that the state had provided to them when they were young, the things that Thatcher's government took away. They operationalized this lived and imagined experience in their understandings of the present and their demands of the future, often referring back to these three time periods to construct their arguments and make sense of what was happening now.

In social movements studies, a life-course approach suggests that retired people are more likely to become involved in political activism because they have more time (Beyerlein and Bergstrand, 2013: 137). Free from the confines of employment, they also have more freedom. They don't need to worry about what the boss might think if she sees them protesting. But the life-course approach does not explain why these particular people got involved in these particular campaigns. Was it because older people need the NHS more? Members of Dunning KONP were – on the whole – quite healthy, only rare users of the NHS, and barely users of other state welfare services. They had mostly retired from professional roles in public services, they owned their own houses, and they lived in one of the more affluent suburbs of Greater Manchester. They were not the population that was most vulnerable in the face of cuts. The impetus towards action was not just personal interest, but also moral outrage at the endangerment of the interests of UK residents in general, and the most vulnerable of UK residents in particular.

In the next section, I explore the life stories of two of the activists that I saw every Tuesday morning: Lily and Leroy. Their narratives demonstrate how it was in the contexts of their own life histories that the aforementioned three time periods overlapped, giving shape to the sense of wrongness that they felt in NHS reforms. By attending to what they saw as morally wrong with the plans for NHS reforms, I search not just for what they objected to, but also an implicit notion of what they understood a good society would look like.

Lily and Leroy

On 30 June 2018, several thousand people[5] marked the 70th anniversary of the NHS by marching through London to protest NHS cuts and privatization. Among these people were me, my family and some of my friends from medical school. We met up with members of Greater Manchester KONP and Dunning KONP. At the next Greater Manchester KONP meeting, we reported on the event and offered various possible explanations for why there were not more people, considering several media outlets were reporting that the NHS was experiencing the worst crisis of its history. Perhaps it was because the Labour Party and the various unions did not organize support well enough or loudly enough. Perhaps it was because it was union conference season, so people's weekends were busy. Perhaps it was because it was summer, so some people were away, and others were just enjoying the sun. Perhaps it was because Prime Minister Theresa May had announced more funds for the NHS just before the march. Or perhaps people were a bit 'marched out'. The week before had seen a march against Brexit, the week after there was to be a march to protest the visit of then American President, Donald Trump, to the UK.

Clearly, NHS activism was not taking place in a vacuum. There was plenty of other stuff going on, some of which was also pretty important. Members of KONP used their own memories to frame and interpret these events in particular ways. After the Greater Manchester KONP meeting, I joined in a conversation between two members, Leroy and Debbie, in which they voiced their worries about the current political moment. Debbie, a retired social worker, said, 'This is the worst time I can remember. This is worse than Thatcher'. Leroy nodded and replied, 'I'm filled with dread. Brexit is awful'. Meanwhile, I overheard two other members, Lily and Ruth, discussing the rise of far-right movements, 'We need to be really careful. There are echoes with the rise of fascism in the 1930s. It's frightening'.

Lily and Leroy were members of Dunning KONP. They also regularly attended meetings of Greater Manchester KONP, seeing themselves as conduits between the two groups, allowing co-operation and facilitation of group activities. I saw them at Greater Manchester KONP meetings, Dunning KONP meetings and at the weekly Dunning KONP protests. I would also often bump into them at protests and marches for climate change, anti-racist events and other causes. During conversations they often explained how these ostensibly unrelated issues were in fact deeply connected. They saw it as their responsibility to participate in all of these movements, as well as some others, often feeling guilty if they missed events.

Lily was 56 years old, making her one of the youngest of the group. Leroy, her partner, was born in 1949. He proudly told me he was one of the first 500,000 babies born in the NHS.[6] He grew up in a suburb of Dunning, in 'the worst kind of housing', a damp, terraced house with an outside toilet and no bathroom. His family lived there until 1956, when the council rehoused the family into what Leroy remembers as 'an incredible house' with running water, electricity and an indoor bathroom. He described his background as poor and working class, as did Lily, who grew up in a small town in Yorkshire. Both of them attended state comprehensive schools and then universities, benefiting from free higher education. Leroy went to art school in Liverpool, whereas Lily trained to become a teacher, thus setting them both up for reasonably well-paid careers which allowed them to buy a large home in Dunning, which was where I interviewed them.

Neither had been politically active until retirement. Lily had worked as a chemistry teacher and head of department, and Leroy had been a graphic designer working at various private companies, and then taught design at a further education college. In 2012, they were among many people that attended a public meeting organized by two other residents of Dunning, Galen and Iris. Iris, a retired social worker, convened the meeting to organize local opposition to the Health and Social Care Bill. Her husband, Galen, a retired professor of medicine and health service manager, spoke about the predicted negative consequences of the bill. The people at the meeting discussed what to do, and decided to form a local group, Dunning KONP. By the time I joined the group in 2017, many members were part of a core that had remained fairly constant since that first meeting in 2012. A few people had dropped out due to illness, time commitments or disagreements with the direction taken by Dunning KONP.[7]

Lily and Leroy had remained very active members of the group. It was often Lily and Leroy that would report back to Dunning KONP meetings on council, clinical commissioning group or trust meetings, having attended to listen and ask questions themselves. Other Dunning KONP members often referred to Lily as one of the most dedicated and passionate members as a result of the research that she did. Lily would normally be quite vocal in meetings, describing what she had heard, read and learnt to others. Leroy would sit back and nod while Lily was speaking, occasionally muttering, 'Yes, yes'. He also helped with graphic design tasks. Leroy designed the website and most of the posters and banners, often with the help of another member, Tony,[8] if there was something that needed to be made by hand. And he would chip in with jokes; spontaneous one-liners offered with a barely veiled smile.

When Lily reported back to meetings, she often referred to issues that were not directly related to the NHS, arguing that 'everything is connected'. They expanded more on this when I interviewed them together. They told me that learning about what was going on in the NHS had spurred them to get involved in other political campaigns. They had joined a branch of the Unite union that was meant for people out of work due to unemployment or retirement. They joined another anti-austerity network in Dunning, with whom they attended the Dunning Job Centre on a weekly basis to campaign against the increasingly punitive measures taken by the Department for Work and Pensions on people who required welfare payments. They spoke very passionately about joining campaigns against fracking and Brexit.

In their eyes, the connection between all of these political issues was austerity, with the crisis in the NHS serving as a symbolic measure of just how deeply consequential the effects of austerity were. In our interview, Leroy told me, 'We see everything as the same problem. Everything goes back to the change of government'. He was referring to the election of the Conservative government in 2010. Telling me about Michael Moore's film, *Sicko* (2007), he added that 'the NHS is shown as a shining example of state-provided healthcare. All the staff are happy, they have enough money to do what they want.' He contrasted Michael Moore's depiction of UK healthcare with 2018, with regular media reports of worsening NHS crisis: worse outcomes for patients, increasing stress for health professionals. Lily replied, 'Everything to do with health, but also everything to do with everything goes back to 2010'. That is, the degradation of healthcare was emblematic of a wider process. We went on to discuss the consequences of cuts to welfare services for the people that they met at job centres. For Lily and Leroy, cuts and privatization in the NHS were metonyms for cuts and privatization in all public services since 2010, when the Tory and Liberal Democrat coalition came to power.

But Lily and Leroy did not form their judgements of the coalition government's actions in isolation. They made comparisons to other periods, using their own experiences as a moral baseline. They compared their own lives – which they considered to be fortunate, happy lives – to the lives of people who were now not being supported by state services in the ways they had been. This included the unemployed or precariously employed people they met at the Job Centre, but also Lily's daughter, Olivia, who was 21 years old.

Olivia had paid tuition fees to attend university and taken out a student loan. Whereas Lily had finished university with a small amount of money still left in the bank, Olivia had finished with a debt of £47,000, which would have been more had Lily not paid some of it off. And whereas Lily had quickly moved into fairly stable work, Olivia had struggled with a variety of insecure and poorly paid jobs, with extremely stressful working conditions. Lily told me of her sadness when Olivia said to her, 'Mum, you have to accept that I will never own a house'.

They attributed the differences in fortunes between Lily and Olivia to changes in society that were partially explained by the different roles of state organizations and private companies in their lives. Lily and Leroy did not pay for their higher education. Lily joked that, due to her student grant, she had finished university with more money than when she started. They believed that they had been able to lead stable, relatively flourishing lives as a result of the free state education they received. They contrasted their own experience with Olivia's, attributing her recent tribulations to having to pay for her higher education, resulting in her being in debt afterwards. They told me that the Student Loans Company was not a state institution; 'the recovery of student debt has been privatized'.[9] This led Leroy back again to how everything was connected, pointing out how privatization had, 'so many times' led to bad outcomes for the individuals using any state services that were now in private hands.

Their pragmatic and moral judgements of policies used their own past memories as a benchmark against which to compare current events, thus forming a narrative of the withdrawal of pre-existing obligations. Withdrawal of a state service was equated with abdication of collective responsibility. They remembered the poverty of their youth as a time of solidarity signified by the support offered them by the state, support that had beneficial effects on their lives. As Leroy said, 'I appreciate what was given to me by the welfare state, by Attlee's incredible government … it's unbelievable what that government achieved. I didn't realize it at the time.' His final sentence indicates how these were judgements he had not come to while growing up, but more recently, after the financial crash, after they witnessed similar state services changing for Olivia, and also for the other people they were meeting as a result of their political activism.

The ways in which the state provided services for citizens in need was significant not just for practical evaluations of how the economy worked, but also shaped Lily and Leroy's interpretations of society itself. They understood evidence of the state's abandonment of the people that they met as a societal abdication of responsibility, for which they felt ashamed. State, society, morality and economy were not separate spheres, but were all intertwined. Their shame – the way they *felt* – shows how they scaled down the state's renunciation of its obligations to their own personal consciences, to be scaled back up through political activism to save the NHS.

They charted the progression from post-war social solidarity to post-crash state negligence by way of a major protagonist in their political memories: Margaret Thatcher. Thatcher's infamous pronouncement that 'there is no such thing as society' hung in the background of their perceptions of political history. They interpreted Thatcher's changes to the state machinery and its services in relation to Thatcherite views that the state should create space for enterprizing, hard-working individuals, rather than care for vulnerable communities. Implicit in Lily and Leroy's reading was that shared ties within such communities were actually broken by Thatcher's approach rather than strengthened. Conversely, state welfare did not lead to a 'dependence culture' or the relinquishing of individual responsibility for oneself, but instead signified and also produced a society in which people were able to take responsibility for one another. For Leroy, this kind of society was what he called 'socialism … the social fabric' tying us together, as opposed to the 'apes around the watering hole' of Thatcher's 'me, me, me society'.

It was the relinquishing of ties between people, the refusal of people to take responsibility for the less well-off that particularly distressed them. Most weeks, Leroy would complain about Brexit to me at the Tuesday morning protests. They had both spent time before the referendum campaigning for Remain, and Leroy had been surprised and deeply upset by the responses of the people in the area in which they lived, largely populated by affluent, white British people of a similar age to them. Many of them voiced concerns about migration and migrants to Leroy, which led him to consider them racist. Aware that it was a Tory constituency, and comparing their views on migrants to the views he assumed they had on austerity, he described his moral outrage. He was angry that they, having grown up at a similar time to him, would have benefited from many free state services that they were now suggesting should be withdrawn from UK citizens and people who wished to move to the UK. Leroy felt that this was hypocritical and mean-spirited, evidence of the worst aspects of the 'me, me, me society', the remains of the post-Thatcher neoliberal era that had only worsened following the financial crash. The state was withdrawing its support for people because 'Thatcher's children' – themselves beneficiaries of such support – were taking it away.

The time periods that Lily and Leroy described did not just happen one after the other. They built on one another. David Cameron and George Osborne's austerity consolidated changes to the state that started with Thatcherism, making 2018 the 'worst time I can remember … worse than Thatcher'. This was worse than Thatcher because, in terms of the effects of Thatcher on state and society, she was still here. 'Thatcher's children'[10] were now in charge! Dunning KONP members remembered the industries either destroyed or privatized by Thatcher. Lily had grown up in a village with a pit at the end of her road, and her grandfather had been a miner who died of silicosis. She remembered the euphoria and the eventual disappointment of the miners' strikes. Other retired members of Dunning KONP and Greater Manchester KONP did not have such close connections to that particular political struggle, but they did all remember Thatcher and the kind of political battles she signified.

It was in relation to Thatcher that the outlines of the iconicity of the NHS become easier to trace. Activist discourse – both in conversation and in literature such as leaflets, articles and books – often traced the beginnings of NHS cuts and privatization to Thatcher's government. Another activist in central Manchester, Nancy, who was just about to retire when I interviewed her, pointed out to me in an interview that Thatcher had intended to fully privatize the NHS. In Nancy's telling, two or three health ministers failed to put forward a convincing plan for privatization, so Thatcher sacked them, eventually appointing Kenneth Clarke. In Nancy's words, Clarke told Thatcher, 'You can't do it. The public will hang you from a lamp-post … What you can do is this, this and this', by which Nancy meant the process of fragmentation which activists often construed reforms from the 1980s to be. She continued, '[Kenneth Clarke] said, "That will set the steps for another Tory government going further later". Which is exactly what it did do.'[11]

In the narrative of NHS activists, Thatcher's politics set up a process in which *all* state welfare services were sold off to private companies, undermining the social ties people had to one another in the country. However, the NHS stood out in that it was so loved by the public that for Thatcher to privatize it, she would have to employ clandestine tactics that would take a long time to pay off. If state services signified the collective responsibility between citizens of the postwar era, then the NHS was the one remnant of that period of time that Thatcher could not completely destroy. However, she could make it vulnerable, so that in the more recent, voluble age of austerity, the NHS was placed at existential risk.

So the NHS does not just serve as a metonym for cuts and privatization in all public services since 2010, but also symbolizes the values of the kind of society that activists imagined Attlee's government to be attempting to create, *and* that such values can be realized. That is, a society in which people care and take responsibility for one another, as evidenced by the ongoing existence of a state that provides services for its residents, even if it is has been diminished. As Leon, the chair of Greater Manchester KONP told me, 'It's there'.

A symbol of socialism

Lily and Leroy provide particularly clear examples of the way that many NHS activists formed their moral arguments in relation to their own memories, providing a narrative that unified several overlapping periods of time in their own life stories. But their stories and arguments were typical among Dunning KONP and Greater Manchester KONP members,[12] who mostly considered themselves 'children of the NHS', and considered the NHS a 'symbol of socialism'.

By bringing into view the memories at play in NHS activists' moral arguments, I have sketched the contours of what they imagine there *ought* to be, incorporating many elements of what there used to be. It was important to save the NHS, because the NHS, as they imagined it, symbolized the kind of state that a good society – a socialist society – should have. The NHS, the state and society in which the activists lived had all undergone huge changes over the courses of their lives. It is in their moral arguments that a particular symbolic view of the NHS comes into sight. Similarly, the NHS as a symbol of socialism brings a particular representation of the state into view.

When I asked activists about what socialism meant to them, they rarely mentioned the state, its structure or who owned the means of production. Instead, they spoke about society, community and collective responsibility. However, insofar as they considered that the NHS was the pre-eminent 'symbol of socialism', it is clear that they considered that the state – here represented by a huge state institution – was a key player in the production and reproduction of such a society. Their memories of a past NHS were powerful because they facilitated an understanding not just of what a good state ought to provide, but also what it could provide. Free, comprehensive, universal healthcare was not just morally desirable. It was politically possible. The NHS's ongoing existence, the fact that it was still 'there', confirmed that the state could continue to provide such services. The picture described by Lily and Leroy was one of national moral degradation, in which the ongoing existence of the NHS represented hope of regeneration.

But how did they square the continuity of the NHS with the fact that the NHS was changing? Healthcare continued to be provided by the NHS, and activists continued to project their memories of what it had provided in the past into their aspirations for what it should provide in the future. They used imagination and memory as tools to make better futures. As social psychologist, Seamus Power (2018: 232) puts it, 'Imagination is one process used to articulate moral societies and to actualize them. These visions of the future are grounded in imagined interpretations of past blueprints for … society.' Even if the NHS had changed and continued to do so, even if what was there was in some ways unrecognizable from what had been, activists' moral arguments stabilized a particular notion of the good society, and the role of the state in such a society, ordered around the NHS. Their descriptions and aspirations for continuity were, in fact, a response not to change *per se*, but to the particular changes that they perceived in the NHS, in society and in the state.

They understood the changes to which they were responding as antithetical to the values of the NHS, and of socialism: 'Everything to do with health, but also everything to do with everything'. The focus on the NHS as a key icon of the socialist worldview was a direct rejoinder to what Dunning KONP members saw as a Tory ideology based on a belief that state interventions could only ever corrupt individual responsibility. Although such an ideology may have been personified in Thatcher, its importance now stemmed from its enthusiastic execution by Tory governments since 2010. Thatcher was the bogeywoman, but ongoing Thatcherism was the real problem. In contrast to their memories of Thatcher and their perceptions of more recent Prime Ministers, NHS activists believed there *was* such a thing as society, and the NHS symbolized not just collective responsibility, but how a state intervention could and should contribute to strengthening and implementing that responsibility. NHS services did morally approvable acts *and* functioned effectively. The NHS was *good*, in both senses of the word.

If the changes against which activists used the NHS as a tool of contestation were particular ones, so were the continuities that the NHS represented in the eyes of activists. Lily and Leroy referred to the postwar welfare state through references to provisions of services for all. Whereas the NHS has been described by some as a national*ist* institution working towards exclusionary, restrictive goals (Cowan, 2020), the activists with whom I spent time did not spontaneously mention the welfare state's connections to colonial exploitation (El-Enany, 2020), or its historical exclusions based on ethnicity (Simpson, 2018) or gender (Pedersen, 2018).

However, when I mentioned problematic aspects of the NHS's past, activists did not deny these past exclusions, nor indeed the ongoing persistence and proliferation of exclusionary boundaries in provision of care (Potter, 2015; Potter et al, 2017; Kang, Tomkow and Farrington, 2019; Tomkow, 2019; Younis and Jadhav, 2019; 2020; Tomkow et al, 2020). As I will explore in later chapters, activists used their partial description of the NHS as a symbolic tool with which to contest those boundaries.[13] They chose particular memories and representations that were targeted according to their ethical worldview, to construct an icon which they could use in a political battle. Leroy handed me a DVD of the film, *Sicko*, and asked me why the NHS was not doing now what it used to do then.

Interpretive battle: what did the example mean?

In 1989, anthropologist Faye Ginsburg published a book now considered to be a classic ethnography of social movements. She spent months with American activists campaigning on the issue of abortion. What was novel about Ginsburg's work was that she spent time with the groups on either side, both the pro-choice activists and the people who call themselves pro-life. She found that both groups considered themselves to be feminists, upholding the value of their own versions of what it meant to be a woman. They were locked in with what Ginsburg refers to as an 'interpretive battle' (1989: 96), in which abortion clinics became 'interpretive battlegrounds' (1989: 97). By this, she meant that both sides contested the meanings of symbols and concepts such as gender, femininity and motherhood, while articulating their moral positions. Thus both sides were able to describe themselves as feminists, while contesting what it meant to be a woman, and what aspects of femininity they were protecting or celebrating through their activism. In so doing, they attempted to define what a woman was. So the battle over abortion rights became a battle over meaning and interpretation.

Thus far I have argued that NHS activists like Lily and Leroy used the NHS as an example of socialist values to contest changes to public policy that they viewed as morally wrong. The wrongness of the policies derived from their contribution to the creation of a society in which people were not taking responsibility for one another. For Robbins (2015), the ritual was the archetypal model for a moral example. Within the special circumstances afforded to a ritual, set back from the hurly-burly of everyday life, a value could be fully realized in a way that would otherwise be unrealistic. Unlike Robbins, I have argued that the case I have described, of the NHS as a moral example, carries its force precisely because Lily and Leroy conceived of it as an example of the state fulfilling its obligations to its citizens, and citizens taking responsibility for one another, in the absence of special circumstances.

Lily and Leroy's political intervention – the precise way in which they made the moral political – relied on a particular meaning of the NHS, one that I have described through their life histories. But, as I have indicated with reference to projects of nationalism and exclusion, Lily and Leroy's understanding of the NHS was not the only one available. They were locked in an interpretive battle. Describing Dunning KONP's campaigns as an interpretive battle highlights how it was not just NHS services that were at stake; the use of the NHS as a moral example placed the meaning of the example itself at risk as well. Activists were using their memories of the NHS not just to make moral sense of what is happening now, but also to make a political *intervention* in the present. They were using the iconography of the NHS in a battle, the contours of which will remain the focus of the remaining chapters of this book.

Here I draw on two anthropologists of ethics: Cheryl Mattingly (2014a; 2014b) and James Laidlaw (2014), to explore the implications of using a moral example in this way, as an intervention in the real world. Robbins' model of the ritual protected the example from the risk of interpretive battle by placing it outwith the social and political forces of everyday life. Thus, according to Robbins, the meaning of the values realized by the example are not in question, they are simply 'in play' for the people who observe or participate in rituals. Mattingly (2014a; 2014b) and Laidlaw (2014) refer to exemplars rather than examples, but in a similar vein to Robbins, meaning resources which people are able to use in their own lives to grasp their own values, fashioning their own ethical selves in the process. While Mattingly and Laidlaw's accounts share many similarities with one another, Mattingly calls on Laidlaw to focus less on 'schooling' or 'pedagogical aspects of developing an ethical self' (Mattingly, 2014a: 479). She notes how Foucauldian accounts such as his 'place great emphasis on preexisting practices, techniques, and models for living. This vocabulary directs our gaze to the features of moral life that are already in place, the technologies that are available to be mastered, the teachers who are there to mentor' (Mattingly, 2014a: 479). Instead, she describes exemplars as resources with which people can conduct experiments and learn from the results. Her examples are tools used to intervene in a 'scene of everyday moral perplexity' (2014a: 484), in which there is a problem that requires attention. Thus she describes situated, practical and action-based solutions to moral puzzles, from which people learn, so that their ethical selves evolve. The examples mutate, and the resources available to actors expand, as their deliberations also become resources to make use of in the future. The grounds of experimentation and deliberation are continually shifting. It may seem obvious that using a tool to change societal structures may lead to changes in those structures; that is the point of political activism. But Mattingly also alerts us to how using exemplars in this way opens up the likelihood of change of the exemplar itself, and contestation over its meaning.

The cases that Mattingly depicts often involve families that have been affected by structural factors that make them more vulnerable than others to suffering. However, they seldom engaged in the kind of contentious politics that Dunning KONP did. In contrast, members of Dunning KONP were mostly white and in relatively comfortable financial situations, even if they had been born into more deprived circumstances than those in which they now lived. But since 2010, they had been witnesses to a society in which they felt that people were no longer looking after one another. They used the NHS as an exemplar through which they could grasp the moral import of what they perceived to be the state's abandonment of its – and society's – obligations to its citizens.

Mattingly's portrayal of exemplars as resources to be used in experiments keeps our eyes open to the contingency of how those exemplars might be interpreted, and what effects such interventions might have when deployed. The meaning of the NHS that took shape in Lily and Leroy's ethical imagination was far from universal. Politicians, cognizant of the iconicity of the NHS, have also waded into the fray, attempting to co-opt its valence to their own ends. In 2010, David Cameron claimed that the Conservative Party were the 'party of the NHS', adding 'I'll cut the deficit, not the NHS'. He then oversaw Andrew Lansley's Health and Social Care Act. After the Act passed through parliament, NHS trusts were instructed to make £22 billion of savings between 2014 and 2022, and Cameron's governments severely constrained funding for the NHS, albeit not as much as they did for other public services. More recently, in 2021, then Secretary of State for Health and Social Care, Matt Hancock, outlined his plans for the NHS to be the 'best health system in the world'. Earlier that year, his department had launched a contact-tracing organization to combat spread of COVID-19. Although the organization was separate from the health service, with many of its functions outsourced to private companies, it was notably named 'NHS Test and Trace'. Similarly, testing centres were branded with the NHS kitemark but run by a variety of outsourced companies. Then Prime Minister, Boris Johnson, described NHS Test and Trace as 'world-beating'.

It did not beat COVID-19. NHS Test and Trace did not avert the second or third national lockdowns, nor a larger number of local lockdowns, not to mention thousands of avoidable deaths before the UK's vaccination campaign (National Audit Office, 2020b; 2021; Calvert and Arbuthnott, 2021).

Cameron's duplicity during my fieldwork and Johnson and Hancock's grandiosity during the pandemic were the subject of much activist commentary. But they are not the key point here. Instead, I want to highlight what the NHS was symbolizing in their discourse. My research was not with Conservative politicians, so my interpretations of their discourse are speculative. Clearly, they did not endorse the NHS as an example of actually existing socialism. For Cameron, the health service was an economic burden, but he signalled that he recognized its social importance. So his brand of Conservatism was supposedly willing to support the NHS. He could thus sell the Tory Party as safe stewards of the economy, able to protect a symbol of national pride by making difficult but necessary cuts to other public services. For Hancock and Johnson, the NHS – including private companies branded with its kitemark – was a demonstration of British superiority and their government's efficacious performance in the face of an unprecedented global crisis. Without examining these interpretations too much here,[14] I merely point out that the activists' interpretation of the NHS was not the only one available. There were interpretive battles going on over what the NHS was. So when they claimed the NHS as the symbol of their political vision, this was the battleground they entered.

Is NHS activism conservative?

Well, activists certainly are often on the defensive. And they did often romanticize institutions and services as they used to exist. But in this chapter, my analysis hasn't stopped there. One of the benefits of ethnographic fieldwork is having the time to get to know people for longer. By spending more time, by digging a bit deeper, I got to learn what saving the NHS – as an example of actually existing socialism – meant to activists. They spoke of the past not because they were dwelling there, ignoring the present. They were appropriating and working on the past to make sense of the present, in an attempt to define and shape our state institutions in the future.

Members of Dunning KONP considered their own ethical and political projects within the contexts of their life histories. They considered themselves 'children of the NHS', people who benefited from state welfare, growing up in a society in which state services were one example of how members of society took responsibility for one another. Margaret Thatcher began a process in which the state gradually withdrew its services, and a 'me, me, me society' developed, one predicated on individual rather than collective responsibility. The NHS served as an example of one such state service being withdrawn. The NHS was important because it worked, and because it still exists, even if it is different to what it once was.

NHS activists did not only consider themselves socialists. They considered the NHS as an example of socialism, one that existed in the real world. Indeed, this was often one of the first things they would tell me when I met them; that the NHS was an example of socialism, and that was why we must save it. Their ethics and politics cohered around their imagination of the NHS. Their imagination of the past and future NHS was a moral cornerstone of their evaluations of the political present, key to understanding their praxis, which I will explore in subsequent chapters.

2

Defending the Indefensible: How Did We Get Here?

In October 2017, I arrived at Wigan Infirmary for an interview with a senior manager. The email from the manager's secretary said to come to car park C at the hospital site and ring the buzzer. When I got there, I rang the buzzer. Nobody answered. People were waiting behind me and shouting. I rang again. Still no answer. I lost my nerve and chose to look for another spot in the main car park and just pay for it. There were no spaces, just drivers in cars waiting in various parts of the car park, poised to snap up any spaces that became vacant. So I went back to car park C. Still no answer. Eventually I went to car park B, which abutted car park C. Someone answered immediately and let me in.

Clearly, the problem was that the first intercom had not been working. What was notable regarding the incident was the utter unsurprisingness of it. I did not mention it to the receptionist when I got to the manager's office, nor to the manager himself. I forgot about it until I got home and began to write my fieldnotes.

The consequences of a lack of resources have been normalized. Often we laugh about it. In 2021, when I had returned to clinical work after completing my doctoral research, a consultant psychiatrist told me the story of the time her office was invaded by bees from a hive that had sprung up outside her window. She couldn't shut the window as it was broken. She attempted to call Facilities. The phone wasn't working as a pipe had leaked through the ceiling onto the phone. She called it, 'Peak NHS'.

More often, it is not funny. Each clinician can tell their own stories of how cuts have affected patients and staff in their own specialty in recent years. Gavin Francis (2023) has written a moving book narrating the problems in general practice. In my field, psychiatry, I have seen patients in outpatient clinics who had not been seen since having been referred by their GP over a year previously. In the emergency department, every time a patient consents to admission to an inpatient mental health ward, the practitioner is obliged to explain to them that they may be waiting hours or even days for the bed to become available. When the patient is eventually transferred to the ward, it may be several hours travel away, making visits from family extremely difficult. If it is located in the same town or city, it may be in a private hospital, alongside self-pay patients, because NHS wards are full.

Clinicians have become habituated to all of this. Systems and the workers in those systems have adapted to figure out ways to reduce the harm caused by such restrictions of resources.[1] Eliminating the harm is no longer an option. For example, providing care for people on trolleys in corridors – rather than bays or rooms, with all the associated space, monitoring and equipment – is now the norm. Corridors are now known as 'temporary escalation spaces'. Despite the word, 'temporary', they run around the year. Hospitals have adapted by allocating staff to be corridor nurses, attempting to maintain oversight in these areas where patients could easily be forgotten or overlooked.

A recent survey by the Royal College of Nursing (2025) highlighted the issue of corridor care and its consequences for patients. Another recent report, commissioned by the incoming Labour government after winning a landslide general election in July 2024, described the NHS as being 'in critical condition' (Darzi, 2024: 11). The narrative being constructed by these reports is one of decline: from a functional to a dysfunctional NHS. This was a narrative that mirrored what activists were telling me in 2017, that the NHS was deteriorating and that patients were suffering as a result. They worried that their message was not getting through to a wider public. The annual NHS satisfaction survey suggests otherwise. The most recent results were the worst ever for public satisfaction with the NHS (Jefferies et al, 2024). Despite this discontent, a majority of the public continue to believe that the NHS should remain available to everyone (82%), free of charge (91%) and primarily funded through taxes (82%).

These competing narratives – of discontent with the service at the same time as agreement with some of its perceived underlying principles – presented a dilemma for activists. They sought to 'save' the NHS. But what was it that they were so keen to protect? A failing health service with deteriorating outcomes? A skeleton service for those unable to afford private insurance? A brand or kitemark obscuring the diversion of public money into private equity? As Colin Lorne and Michael Lambert put it, 'When was the NHS?' (2023: 62), and 'Where is the NHS?' (2023: 65). Lorne and Lambert challenge activists to put more meat on the bones of their critique. Which NHS did they want to defend? They highlight the dangers of such narratives of decline, if they remain unqualified, since they could imply that what existed before (whether that is the NHS of 1948 or the NHS of 2010) was good enough.

Activists were acutely aware of their dilemma. The basic story as they saw it was: a once great institution that catered for broad social need has been consistently attacked from the 1980s onwards, with disastrous consequences for quality and comprehensiveness of care. But how could they criticize the problems to which they objected while also supporting what they valued about the NHS? Pretty much every meeting I attended involved at least one discussion related to this question. As Galen, the retired professor of medicine, put it at one meeting of Dunning Keep our NHS Public: 'They are trying to get us to defend the indefensible'.

This quotation points to multiple layers of the work that activists were doing, which will be explored throughout this book. His use of the word, 'They', indicates not just decline, but also purposeful destruction by a malign other. Subsequent chapters will explore this personification and other aspects of how narratives were mobilized by activists, with what consequences, particularly for understanding the political ethics of NHS activism and the group formations that were engendered. This chapter focuses on the content of the narrative itself, and the policy and budgetary background behind it. While staying close to the activist narrative, I will also indicate where other narratives have butted up against it or contradicted it. Moreover, and key to Lorne and Lambert's concerns, I will highlight where nationalist narratives have co-opted the language of defending 'our NHS'. As historian Andrew Seaton (2023) and political scientist Liam Stanley (2022) have outlined, the politics of the 'hostile environment' has a long lineage in relation to the NHS, which I will locate in the history of British colonialism.

Although this chapter focuses on policies, it is important to remember that these policies did not *begin* with governments, just as the history of the NHS did not begin in 1948. The state actors discussed below were all embedded in social and historical environments to which they were crafting their own responses. Attlee and Bevan were living in a 'revolutionary moment' (William Beveridge, quoted by Shore and Wright, 2011: 1), responding to various social factors including the upheaval of war, a landslide Labour election victory, the wild popularity of the Beveridge Report, the organization and activism of socialist groups such as the Socialist Medical Association and the opposition of professional groups such as the British Medical Association.

Nor did the policies that inaugurated the NHS *end* in 1948. Each policy intervened in the social environment in a way that took on its own history, to be interpreted and mobilized in different ways by different actors over time. It is these interpretations that will breathe life into the events described in this chapter, demonstrating how policies and outcomes fragment as people use them to tell different stories with divergent purposes and consequences. Lily and Leroy used their memories of the 'unbelievable' achievements of 'Attlee's incredible government' to tell a story of unfair and uneven retrenchment of state services. They *used* that story to put pressure on today's government. But they were going up against other stories, other memories, other interpretations of policies and, indeed, of the NHS itself.

While this chapter focuses on the activist narrative of decline, later chapters will describe what happened when they took their narratives into political battles to save the NHS.

Like Lily and Leroy, many activists saw the history of the NHS as split into two main sections: before 2010 and after 2010. In this chapter I have followed their template.

Before 2010: the birth of the NHS

The NHS has existed since 1948, when an already existing network of independent, charity and military hospitals were combined under state control, under the aegis of Labour Prime Minister, Clement Attlee, and Minister of Health, Aneurin Bevan (Webster, 2002). It has been described as a 'fundamental component of social solidarity and equal citizenship for over sixty years' (Leys and Player, 2011: ix), an account that fits with Lily and Leroy's understandings of the postwar period. Such a description implies consensus regarding support for the NHS. However, as Andrew Seaton's recent history, *Our NHS* (2023), describes, support has never been unanimous. Although the narrative of the NHS being a result of working-class struggle is popular, Seaton's book adds texture to this story. There were many struggles, arguments and counter-arguments, not just between classes but within them. Importantly, these struggles have evolved over the years, as did the narratives they adopted, moulding and being moulded by actors and movements according to their interests as they perceived them at particular historical conjunctures.

It is a commonplace to hear of the opposition of doctors, manifested by the British Medical Association (henceforth BMA, the main professional association and trade union for doctors in the UK), and the material consequences of such opposition. Aneurin Bevan 'stuffed their mouths with gold' to get them to agree to work in the NHS. Doctors working at consultant level became – and still are – the best paid clinical professionals in hospitals. In addition, they retained the ability to supplement their income with private work.

But doctors were not the only people that had to be convinced. The sustenance of the NHS has been an ongoing project undertaken by its champions, in the face of – at times vociferous – opposition. There has always been a central ethical core linked to its political justification, valorization and defence. In 1951, in a statement to the House of Commons Aneurin Bevan said, 'Ever since 1945 we have been engaged in this country in the most remarkable piece of social reconstruction the world has ever seen. By the end of 1950 we had ... assumed the moral leadership of the world' (1951).

MPs on the other side of the house sniggered. Nevertheless, activists making the case for the NHS often incorporated similar moral narratives into their campaigns. Among these activist groups were the Fabian Society and the Socialist Medical Association, a group I will discuss at greater length in Chapter 5. Universalism was a central concern for them. However, for their arguments to hold water took significant effort. The now common narrative of the 'spirit of '48', engendered by the conflict of 1939–1945 in a context of total war, does not tell the whole story.

Seaton (2023) explains the various anxieties that the public had regarding accessing healthcare from a state institution. They were used to accessing healthcare from a family doctor whom they considered to be a part of their community. If they set foot in hospitals, these were often run by charities. Payments were determined by almoners who visited patients to assess what they were able to pay (Gosling, 2018). The public did not yet understand health and healthcare as entitlements or rights. They had to be encouraged to use the 'National Health'. The maintenance of local General Practitioners (GPs, the UK term for family doctors) in their independent practices was one way in which people were persuaded that they would still be treated as individual people, rather than numbers by the state machine.

The contractual arrangements for general practice were a further concession to the BMA. Rather than being directly employed by the NHS, GPs have always been 'independent contractors'.[2] Maintaining these practices as they were before 1948 meant that these were mostly small practices of just one doctor or small partnerships, often in a household setting. The doctors were usually men and it was not uncommon for the doctor's wife to do the cleaning, book-keeping and other tasks, with no separate payment. That is, other than the capitation fees that the doctor received for each patient, the wives were unpaid for their work.

This model developed over the years. Following the Family Doctor Charter of 1966, which addressed GPs' feelings of being overworked and undervalued, working in inappropriate household environments, the Labour government of the 1960s encouraged the development of larger partnerships working out of specially designed health centres. Although there were many advantages to working in more modern premises, it became less common for doctors to be understood as members of the communities in which they worked. Larger partnerships allowed for greater labour flexibility and female GPs became more common. However, seeing the same doctor every time you visited – also known as continuity of care – became less common. Instead, people saw whichever doctor was available.

The colonial backbone of the NHS

The number of female GPs has grown consistently; there are now over 10,000 more women than men (Yang, 2024). The general practice workforce provides an example not just of changing gender dynamics within the NHS, but also the ways in which migrant labour has been encouraged and even relied upon. In his book, *Migrant Architects of the NHS*, Julian Simpson (2018), documents the role that non-UK trained doctors played from 1948 onwards. Experiencing professional discrimination, migrant doctors' career options were limited. Therefore, these doctors became over-represented in areas where other doctors were less willing to work, often industrial areas and inner cities. As a result, he argues that they were key to the core mission of the NHS to provide care for everyone, including less wealthy communities. His book focuses on general practice doctors in the first decades of the NHS, but the story of migrant workers plugging gaps in the NHS workforce persists, is pervasive across all medical specialties and includes many of the non-medical professions, such as nursing, physiotherapy and other technical staff (Mallorie, 2024).

My own family is one example. My father moved to the UK from India in 1981. After struggling to make way in his preferred career of rheumatology, he chose to work as a GP. My mother then arrived with my brother. I was born shortly afterwards and we settled in London, with my father working in one of its most deprived boroughs.

As Simpson documents, in the first instance most of these workers were migrating from places that were formerly British colonies. The British Nationality Act of 1948 had transformed the people living in the Commonwealth from subjects of British Empire to British citizens (Stanley 2022), making migration possible. The Windrush generation were an exemplary case, invited from the Caribbean in the 1950s and 1960s to plug holes in the British workforce. Despite their nominal citizenship, people already living in the UK understood them as 'immigrants'. Hostility to these perceived outsiders grew, leading to the term 'immigrant' becoming racialized. Further changes to the law in 1962 and 1971 added barriers to citizenship that made migration from predominantly black and brown countries more challenging. (For more detailed explorations see El-Enany, 2020; Stanley, 2022; Pushkar and Tomkow, 2025.)

The Windrush generation were later to become among the more flagrantly unjust victims of hostile environment policies.[3] The story of encouraging racialized people from former colonies to come and work in the NHS, only to stigmatize them and treat them less favourably than other employees, demonstrates the imbrication of the British welfare state with its colonial history.[4]

The particular focus that is relevant for this book is that a state service that had been conceived by Bevan as based on 'universality' of access, was being used to consolidate differences between people understood as British and people understood as 'immigrants'. This harnessing of the ethical symbolism of the NHS to a depiction of the nation (and/or state) is one that has figured throughout its history, making the health service rhetorically useful for politicians. The hostile environment and the UK's response to COVID-19 provide particularly egregious recent examples of this 'welfare nationalism' (Seaton, 2023: 6), since they excluded people in the UK who were considered not part of a racialized understanding of the nation. However, movements seeking to 'save the NHS' from privatization have not been immune from their own versions of welfare nationalism, in which the commodification of public services has been rendered as Americanization, unlike the NHS's unique expression of solidaristic British values.

Thatcher and the market

The Thatcher period, from 1979 to 1990, brought a radical reappraisal of welfare policies. Before 1979, groups that opposed state provision of healthcare (such as the Institute for Economic Affairs and the Fellowship for Freedom in Medicine) had been influential within the Conservative Party but had not succeeded in bringing marketization into the NHS (Koram, 2022; Seaton, 2023).[5] Following the economic turbulence of the 1970s, Thatcher's government wanted to reduce government spending and minimize public services provided by the state. But, as Nancy pointed out in Chapter 1, they had to reconcile this desire with the popular prestige of the NHS. Therefore, the Thatcher government remained ostensibly committed to maintaining the original ideals of universality, comprehensiveness and being free at the point of delivery. At the same time it began a process of incremental reforms, each step preparing the way for the next. Meanwhile, leaks of cabinet papers revealed Tory ministers' 'revulsion against statism' (Webster, 2002: 144) and their underlying aim of gradually reconstructing the service on the basis of private insurance.

Thatcher's reforms of the state are often labelled as 'neoliberal', a word used more commonly now than then. The term has been criticized by anthropologists (Eriksen et al, 2015) as being used to describe so many different things in so many different social and political contexts that it becomes meaningless. Often what is being referred to is a reduction in state interventions and expenditure. However, as Quinn Slobodian (2018) has demonstrated, for the economists who coined the term, neoliberalism did not mean *less* state intervention, but instead referred to the kinds of state intervention of which they approved. Specifically, the neoliberal approach to governance favoured active state interventions to create and protect markets in such a way that capitalists could make profits and thus be incentivized to continue investing. Neoliberal thinkers approved of governmental strategies such as subduing unions and suppressing popular protest.[6]

Slobodian's conceptualization of neoliberalism neatly fits Thatcher's government's actions, which included interventions to halt the removal of pay-beds from NHS hospitals and encourage hospital consultants to undertake more private practice. Her government also used personal tax exemptions and town and country planning legislation to boost the growing private health insurance market. But there was also a principled tenor to her approbation of individually focused, self-funded healthcare, as opposed to the shared nature of public healthcare, with its open wards and free access. She used private hospitals herself and chastised her ministers if they used the NHS since it set the wrong example. As Andrew Seaton puts it: 'Thatcher pursued a moral project that sought to foster self-reliance. Accordingly, the Conservatives also aimed to "residualize" the welfare state by making it the crutch of the very poor, rather than a set of services regularly accessed by all Britons' (2023: 207). That is, she was very happy for the state to intervene in the market to encourage exchanges that fit her normative model for the economy.

The Griffiths Report of 1983 is commonly regarded as the first step the government made towards marketization *in* the NHS (Krachler, 2013; Krachler and Greer, 2015). The report was led by the managing director of a large supermarket chain, Sainsbury's. He recommended that general management structures be set up at all levels of the NHS, as well as an NHS Management Board, thus beginning the process of reducing the grip of medical professionals, ministers and civil servants. At the same time, the Department for Health and Social Security issued a directive stating that all ancillary services should be put up for competitive tender, amounting to approximately 12% of the NHS budget. For example, cleaning was one of the first services to be outsourced in the early 1980s (Ormerod, 2018a).[7]

It was at this point, in the 1980s, that campaign groups opposing cuts and privatization, such as London Health Emergency, began to emerge, raise awareness and place pressure on politicians and NHS managers. Between 1948 and the 1980s, promotion of the NHS within the UK was no longer such a pressing concern, so organized campaigns had fallen away. Instead, activism had focused on transforming the care provided *in* the NHS, particularly by accounting for changes in social attitudes, for example regarding sex, gender, ethnicity and relationships. These campaigns drove changes such as allowing parents to stay with their children on paediatric wards, facilitating free access to contraceptive advice, devices and medication, and providing written materials in multiple languages.

In 1963, Helen Hodgson formed the Patients Association. This organization helped to cement British people's conceptualization of themselves as citizens with a right to adequate healthcare. But the language of patient rights also dovetailed with that of consumers. As Seaton writes, 'the patients' movement and consumerism conjoined to empower ordinary people to critique the paternalism of modern medicine' (2023: 90). A notable example of such rights-based activism is the anti-psychiatry movement, which looked to eliminate the human rights abuses of psychiatry, most obviously the right to freedom lost by locking people away in asylums. The campaigns were galvanized throughout the 1960s and 1970s by multiple abuse scandals in the asylums, which were poorly maintained Victorian buildings, generally located outside cities. However, it was not until the 1980s, when the demands of these movements aligned with the Thatcher government's desire to close down large state-led institutions of care, that the Griffiths Report proposed relocating the patients from asylums to smaller locations in communities.

Social care

The closure of the asylums led to a boom in privately run residential care homes, often run by business-minded healthcare professionals who had noticed this new gap in the market. Since this care was still paid for by the state, the change to community care did not save money. However, Thatcher approved of the entrepreneurship demonstrated by these clinicians, as well as the reduced state control, and so personally blocked attempts to limit spending in this area (Lewis and Glennerster, 1996).

The story of social care is closely intertwined with that of the NHS. I only have space for a brief outline (but see Gingrich, 2011; Hayes, 2017; Koch, 2018; Bottery and Jefferies, 2025 for more detail). Social security funding was available from 1948 for those who needed care. The numbers were initially very low.[8] In 1980, the Conservative government introduced a subsidy allowing state support for the poorest people to live in private care homes. A (state-funded) market was thus created, leading to a slew of new, poorly regulated care homes. As the numbers of people eligible for the subsidy rose, the state sought to reduce costs. In 1990, the Conservative government passed the Community Care Act, under which private care services sought contracts from local authorities by competitive tendering.[9]

Local authorities chose not to fund the best possible care for all people. Therefore, wealthier people paid from their own pockets for better care. Costs were shifted onto individuals and their families. Gingrich writes: 'Wealthy users could buy high-quality care at high prices from exclusive private providers, low-income users received public funding for low-quality care, while middle-income users were stuck paying high fees while receiving the same low-quality care as the publicly-funded users' (2011: 184).

When the Labour Party came to power in 1997, they did provide more funding but did not alter the overall model, other than focusing more on 'personalized' services and budgets, in which individuals were 'empowered' to choose the care they needed. Simon Duffy, researcher, activist and founding director of the Centre for Welfare Reform, was a key proponent of the move to personalization. Looking back in 2014, after budgets had been cut back again, he wrote: 'personalisation has become an excuse for abandonment … personalisation has become an excuse to cut costs' (2014).

Today, social care providers are largely privately owned. State funding continues to be from local government. Therefore, when austerity hit, social care was one of the main victims. Funding fell by 55% between 2010 and 2016, at the same time as the population growing older (Curry et al, 2024). Where funding is not provided by the state, costs are met by private spending by individuals. Such costs can be catastrophic. Demand for care has continued to rise. Although funding has increased somewhat since 2016, it has not kept pace with the increasing demand. In addition, social care units are understaffed by insecure, poorly paid workers (Bottery and Jefferies, 2025), often migrants threated by the insecurity of the hostile environment.[10] The situation is commonly described as a crisis (NHS Confederation, 2022). But it has been a crisis in plain view for many years.

The relevance for this book is the impact of inadequate social care on the NHS. When people are admitted to hospital, they cannot be discharged until a place has been found for them that the clinical team consider to be safe for them to go to, with adequate social support. The crisis in social care means that it can take days or weeks for this social support to be arranged. During that time the patient has to stay in that hospital bed, thus reducing the amount of vacant beds for new patients to be admitted. This is widely known as bed-blocking or delayed discharges. Bed-blocking is understood to be one key source of the capacity issues in the NHS, which will be discussed in more detail below. Furthermore, when people are discharged to placements with substandard social care, they are more likely to become unwell again, and require more outpatient care or even readmission to hospital.

The internal market

An internal market was introduced in 1990, in which local health authorities 'purchased' healthcare from hospitals and other 'providers' of care. It was called 'internal' because all of the providers remained a part of the NHS and the funding was still provided by the government. When the Labour Party came to power in 1997, funding increased and there was a sustained effort to recruit and train more staff, leading to 50,000 more doctors and 100,000 more nurses and midwives (Krachler, 2013). But the marketization process continued. Health authorities became Primary Care Trusts (PCTs), which were to commission services from providers of care which were no longer limited to the NHS. Thus an 'entry point' (Krachler and Greer, 2015: 215) for private healthcare was created, to provide care that would be commissioned and paid for by the state, remaining free to the patient.[11]

The entry point was not just created. It was incentivized.[12] To encourage the investment in and development of Independent Sector Treatment Centres (ISTCs), the NHS paid them 11.5% more than the equivalent cost of an operation provided by the NHS. Contractual efforts were also made to reduce the risk that the private sector might not recoup its investment. Block guaranteed payments were made to ISTCs irrespective of whether they undertook the contracted number of procedures for the NHS. The government also agreed that it would buy back some treatment centres at the end of the five-year contracts (Rowland, 2022).

Another source of private investment in UK state public services was Private Finance Initiatives (PFIs). PFIs, pioneered in the UK before being exported to other countries, facilitated short-term injections of capital but were tied to contracts which held public sector organizations – including NHS trusts – in debt to private companies to be paid back at high interest rates over long periods of time. For example, one contract signed by Oxleas NHS Foundation Trust in 1998, will run until 2050.[13]

Although Chancellor of the Exchequer Gordon Brown justified these contracts as a 'sharing of risk' that was in the public interest, in fact it was an appropriation of risk by the state. Once signed, the state had to pay up as stipulated. But if the company failed to deliver, the state still had to step in, or face the possibility of not having a hospital. In 2018, when construction company Carillion collapsed before completing the new Royal Liverpool University Hospital, the government had to provide further funds to complete the project (National Audit Office, 2020a).

Commissioning was a key lever for opening the market to the private sector. But the government did not admit as much. Instead, the government argued that commissioning would improve efficiency. The logic was symmetrical to that of the Washington Consensus's structural adjustment policies in underdeveloped countries: competition breeds efficiency (Basilico et al, 2013). This logic has prevailed for all services in the neoliberal state, not just healthcare. Outsourcing has grown and grown, with private sector involvement heaviest in IT, construction, waste management, building maintenance, social care and defence (Walker and Tizard, 2018).

Outsourcing and state capacity

Specialist NHS services provide discrete nuggets that can be bracketed and parcelled off. For example, more than half of England's sexual assault referral centres are now run by G4S and Mountain Healthcare (which is owned by a private equity group set up by Paul Pindar, former managing director and chief executive of Capita) (Marsh and Garcia, 2024).

Sam Freedman, a former adviser to Tory politician Michael Gove and now writer and think tank researcher, has recently written on the topic of outsourcing in the UK, and its effects on state capacity (2024). For competition to achieve the goal of reducing costs requires certain conditions of a well functioning market: multiple organizations able to provide the relevant service, an easy way to measure and compare the services provided, and accountability for failure to be assumed by the contracted company.

In healthcare, none of the market conditions described by Freedman are met. To use the example of sexual assault referral centres, there are very few organizations that can provide such services in any given town or city. Quality of provision of healthcare generally – and support following sexual assault in particular – is difficult to measure. And if the service fails, the provider has lost nothing (other than possibly the securement of the next contract, although even this loss would rely on the service's failure being recognized by the commissioning body). It is patients and families that suffer. Meanwhile the wider NHS absorbs the cost of that specific service failure. If patients end up more unwell and more in need of care, they attend emergency departments and GP practices more, are more likely to require inpatient admission, and outpatient follow-up will have to be provided by another community team.

Freedman notes that the UK state has not only contracted services out where these conditions are not met. It has become so addicted to contracting out that it has lost the capacity it once had to provide many services. Therefore, the state is locked into a position of *having* to contract out, very often to one of the 'Big Four' who dominate the UK market: Serco, Capita, Atos and G4S. Serco usefully demonstrates the breadth of public service provision dominated by these huge players. Freedman writes that Serco runs detention centres for asylum seekers, facilities management for hospitals, cycle hire schemes in various cities, ferry services to the Orkney and Shetland islands, six prisons, the warning system for incoming nuclear missiles, programmes to help unemployed people back into work, and bin collection in several councils.

If everyone knows that services are being contracted out even when the conditions for a well-functioning market are not being met, why has the UK state continued to outsource? One reason is the aforementioned loss of state capacity. The state has outsourced so many services for so long, that it now simply cannot do otherwise. As such, outsourcing is now less driven by ideology and more by necessity. Economist Daniela Gabor has formulated this development as the evolution from the Washington Consensus to the Wall Street Consensus.[14] In the latter, the state's priority is to encourage private investment. In order to do so, it must de-risk the investment, thus taking on the risk itself. It does so by providing long-term contracts for state services, with no penalties for defaulting on contracts. Thus the organizations able to fund these large investments end up with unparalleled power, able to dictate terms to states without which they will simply invest elsewhere. She writes: 'Having dragged the poor into the embrace of the market [via the Washington Consensus's focus on marketization], financial capital turns to colonizing the infrastructure of the state [via the Wall Street consensus's focus on long-term derisked contracts for essential state services]' (2021: 436).

The NHS and management consultancies

As mentioned, a well functioning market requires the ability to compare different providers of services. Healthcare quality is notoriously difficult to measure and compare. Therefore, at the same time as introducing the internal market, the Labour government attempted to monitor and improve efficiency by introducing various performance indicators. These included the four-hour target, under which trusts aimed for patients attending emergency departments to be admitted, transferred or discharged within four hours of attending (Department of Health, 2000). Trusts were to aim for 97% of patients to meet this target initially. The target was raised to 98% in 2005 (BBC News, 2005).

In some ways, the proliferation of numbers presented a good news story for the Labour government. Waiting lists that had built up during the Conservative governments of Margaret Thatcher and John Major were largely eliminated. Following an outpatient referral by one's GP, most people expected to be seen by a specialist and treated within 18 weeks. The new independent sector treatment centres did play a role in this. However, the vast bulk of backlog-busting between 2000 and 2010 was done by NHS staff being paid extra to work overtime in existing NHS facilities (Dixon, Jones and Mays, 2011; Ham, 2023).

Another consequence of the introduction of performance indicators became apparent after trusts were given the ability to become 'foundation trusts' in 2003. Foundation trusts were financially independent, meaning they were given the ability to borrow money (up to a limit), and to make and keep surpluses. Most importantly, resources could now be allocated by 'payment by results'. How they performed on the relevant indicators contributed to how much money they would receive. Trusts were still owned by the state but were encouraged to think and behave like businesses.[15] They were not just competing with the private sector treatment centres that could now acquire contracts to provide NHS services. NHS trusts were also competing with each other.

I have already mentioned the 'Big Four' public service contractors. Here we move onto another 'Big Four'. Most of the plans that led to the foundation trust reforms were written not just by politicians and civil servants, but also management consultants from the 'Big Four' accountancy firms or the other management consultancy firms that provide similar services (Ormerod, 2018b; Mazzucato and Collington, 2023). The centrality and importance of management consultants led to a 'revolving door' between government, the civil service, NHS organizations and consultancy firms, blurring lines of accountability and leading many people working in the NHS to suspect conflicts of interest (Oliver, 2014) among those charged with making health policy.[16]

As with the Big Four contractors, the legacy of NHS involvement with the Big Four management consultancies is an ever-increasing foothold in the NHS. Mazzucato and Collington (2023), economists whose work focuses on interactions between the public and private sectors, found that NHS spending on management consultants trebled 2016 to 2019. Nevertheless, the involvement of management consultancies has never been displayed to the public. Instead, plans were often presented to the public by senior clinicians, especially doctors, allowing politicians to describe reforms as 'clinically led' (Barker, 2010; Jones and Exworthy, 2015; Jones, 2016).[17]

Changes after 2010: the Health and Social Care Act

David Cameron became Prime Minister in 2010, leading a coalition government of Tories and Liberal Democrats until 2015, when he and the Tories won an outright majority. When he entered office, public satisfaction in the NHS stood at the highest level since records had begun (Park et al, 2012). Cameron, aware of public sentiments, publicly embraced the NHS in a way that previous Conservative politicians had not. In contrast to Thatcher's trumpeting of her own private health insurance plan, Cameron openly discussed his family's use of the NHS. He sought to project an image of his government as one that would not attack the NHS or its values, but instead protect it, albeit according to principles of fiscal discipline, which he and his government rendered as a greater danger than the private sector itself. While campaigning for election, he declared that he would 'Cut the deficit, not the NHS' and that there would be 'no more of the tiresome, meddlesome, top-down re-structures that have dominated the last decade of the NHS'.

Once in power, the coalition government launched what then chief executive of the NHS, David Nicholson, described as 'a reorganisation so big you can see it from outer space' (Cameron, 2014).[18] The Health and Social Care Act was introduced in 2012, under which Primary Care Trusts were replaced by Clinical Commissioning Groups (CCGs), which were now able to purchase services from 'any qualified provider'. The 'any' signified that when CCGs made decisions regarding whom to commission a service from, they should have no regard for whether or not that organization was state-run. This was 'supposed to complete the project of making the NHS more efficient by fragmenting it into a system of independent trusts and subjecting them to market competition' (Leys, 2016: 12).

Trusts were further encouraged to act like businesses, empowered to borrow money and also to pursue profit from private healthcare themselves, up to 49% of their income. Then Secretary of State for Health, Andrew Lansley, explained that he aimed to make changes to the NHS that were 'permanent' (quoted by Timmins, 2018: 12). The purpose, stated explicitly, was to create an NHS that was responsive to market pressures, rather than micro-managed by meddling politicians.[19]

Although the Act (building on the establishment of foundation trusts) encouraged trusts to act *like* private enterprises, there has only been one occasion in which a whole trust was actually privatized. In 2012, a private-equity controlled company, Circle, took over management of an already-existing NHS hospital trust in Cambridgeshire. Its deficit doubled and care quality fell such that the UK's monitoring organization, the Care Quality Commission, rated it as inadequate and placed it under special measures. Circle walked away in 2015 and the NHS was left to pick up the pieces (Leys, 2016).[20]

By 2014, it was widely accepted in NHS management that predictions of failure (e.g. Pushkar, 2012) had been correct. Even Tory politicians recognized the Act's problems, albeit quietly. Andrew Lansley was replaced by Jeremy Hunt as Secretary of State for Health not long after the Act was passed. David Cameron is reported to have regretted the Act (Iacobucci, 2014), and an anonymous Conservative Cabinet minister is quoted by Timmins (2018: 4) as saying it 'was our biggest mistake in government'.

NHS England was one of the bodies newly set up by the Act, to oversee the implementation of policy in the NHS, but at arm's length.[21] When a new chief executive, Simon Stevens, was appointed in 2014, the direction of NHS reforms changed somewhat. He released a plan entitled the *5 Year Forward View* (NHS England, 2014). The document does not mention competition at all, and instead focuses on integration and collaboration. However, at the same time, Stevens had to manage the austere fiscal environment dictated by the Tory government. He instructed trusts to make £22 billion of savings by 2021–2022. In 2016, 44 districts were asked to publish a Sustainability and Transformation Plan (STP), showing how they would integrate services and use 'new models of care' (NHS England, 2014: 30) to make these efficiency savings. Later, in 2017, NHS England proposed Accountable Care Organizations as new bodies that could help integrate health with social care, and NHS management with local government. Chapter 3 will take up the story of Accountable Care Organizations from here.

Devo Manc

The already complex policy and administrative ecology of the NHS was complicated further by the announcement in 2014 that Greater Manchester's most senior local government officials had negotiated a deal for devolution with the Tory national government.[22] The agreement handed over administration of transport, housing and skills budgets as long as Greater Manchester elected a mayor (Walshe et al, 2018). In February 2015, control of healthcare was added. What was negotiated was described as 'devolved control' (Walshe et al, 2018: 9) of the £6 billion per annum budget for health and social care for the 2.8 million people of the city-region.

A new body was set up, the Greater Manchester Health and Social Care Partnership (GMHSCP), led by an employee of NHS England, Jon Rouse. The GMHSCP had representation from the mayor, from each council in Greater Manchester, from each CCG and from each of the NHS trusts that provided care. In December 2015, it published its first strategic plan, *Taking Charge* (Greater Manchester Combined Authority, 2015). Like the *5 Year Forward View*, the document identified the problems of rising demand for healthcare in an increasingly unequal population, at the same time as a rapidly growing 'financial challenge' (Greater Manchester Combined Authority, 2015: 47). The way to solve these problems was by integrating health and social care, NHS and local government, using 'new models of care'.[23]

As already mentioned, the impact of changes to healthcare services is difficult to measure. Available research has suggested that devolution had mixed consequences including some successes. For example, one paper demonstrated that life expectancy and healthy life expectancy rose in Greater Manchester faster than expected (where the expected figure was modelled by a synthetic control) (Britteon et al, 2024).

Immigration

In 2012, the British government outlined plans to decrease net immigration 'from the hundreds of thousands to the tens of thousands' (Travis, 2013). Theresa May, then Home Secretary, said the aim of the plans was to create 'a really hostile environment for illegal migration' (quoted by Kirkup and Winnett, 2012). The Immigration Acts of 2014 and 2016 restricted migrants' welfare and healthcare entitlements. Since then, clinicians and administrative staff have been mandated to monitor people accessing state services and check whether people are 'entitled' to free NHS care (Kang, Tomkow and Farrington, 2019; Tomkow, 2019; Tomkow et al, 2020).

The government's rationale for these changes referred to 'healthcare tourists', people who were coming to the UK specifically to make use of NHS care, at the cost of the UK taxpayer (Pushkar, 2017). In 2017, NHS charging regulations were extended; irregular migrants must now pay before receiving treatment in certain services.[24] The result of hostile environment policies has been restrictions in access to healthcare that have been differentiated not just by nationality, but also by ethnicity. To put it more starkly, people of colour have found it more difficult to access healthcare.[25] The government's summary of its public consultation on charging regulations read, 'the NHS should be a national not an international health service' (Department of Health, 2013, quoted by Lonergan, 2020: 13).[26]

Much has been written on the impacts of Brexit and migration on attitudes, discourse, policy and legislation relevant to the NHS (e.g. Buchan, 2023). What is important for this book is the ways in which the NHS has been employed in these debates. Recent scholarship has worried that 'campaigns to "keep the NHS public" reify a particular nationalistic ideal, bringing about a shared identity which can be exclusionary of those who experience discrimination or other negative experiences within healthcare' (Cowan, 2024: 1153). Hannah Cowan's work[27] clearly demonstrates the ongoing misogyny and racism in the NHS.

Her research was with orthopaedic surgeons and their patients, rather than with activists or others making conscious use of the iconography of the NHS. When Cowan's work is combined with the hostile environment's depiction of the NHS as a fragile jewel in need of protection from the coarse, dirty hands of the outsider, it becomes possible to see how governing parties are utilizing a particular interpretation of the NHS that is at odds with Lily and Leroy's. Theresa May portrayed the Conservative party as on the side of the British people, protecting their interests by first rendering the NHS as under threat from healthcare visitors, and then enacting policies that exclude such visitors. Opposition parties who pander to marginalized groups could thus be portrayed as a soft touch, whose moralizing approach to immigration did not serve the interests of British citizens.[28] It is important to note the racialized understanding of who counts as British implicitly under-writing this narrative. This was welfare nationalism in action. The continuity with what I referred to earlier as the colonial backbone of the NHS is easy to discern.

On the other hand, historians of migration and NHS have noted that the NHS was not just a site of racism and a focus of race-anxiety, but also a site in which antipathy to racism was both effected (through recognition of the contribution of NHS workers, albeit unevenly and inconsistently) and staged (through images, TV dramas, the Olympics opening ceremony) (Bivins, 2015; Crane, 2019). The political campaigns against healthcare charges for migrants are one example of this organizational anti-racism *within* the NHS. The various mobilizations of the NHS to contrary ends speak to its iconicity and its multivalent meanings.

Funding

Welfare retrenchment, more commonly known as austerity,[29] has been common across Northern and Western European countries since the 1970s (Ebbinghaus, 2015), and has accelerated since the financial crash of 2008. As observed by political scientist Tom O'Grady (2022), austerity has not just been dramatically more pronounced in the UK than in the rest of Europe, but also more popular. However, it is well recognized that the cost of healthcare has been rising in the same period (Rodriguez Santana et al, 2020). Therefore, spending on the NHS has risen every year since its inception.[30]

Initially in 1948, the NHS was underfunded when compared to other state services, such as education (Cutler, 2006). Until 1997, the rate of growth was relatively constant, between 3–4%. By 1984, this persistent growth had reversed the comparative underfunding (Seaton, 2023). When Labour won a majority in 1997, they raised spending to levels closer to the Western European average, at 6% growth. When the Tories came to power in the coalition government in 2010, the rate of growth fell dramatically, to around 1% (Charlesworth, Watt and Johnson, 2018).[31]

In this environment of constrained funds, local managers had to find areas to make what the *5 Year Forward View* optimistically called 'efficiency gains' (NHS England, 2014: 36), *Taking Charge* called 'efficiency improvements' (Greater Manchester Combined Authority, 2015: 43), and the National Audit Office called 'efficiency savings' (National Audit Office, 2019: 8).[32]

Alternative sources of funding

In the absence of further funds from central government, managers were driven to raise capital for services through one-off sales that continued the history of loss of publicly-owned assets to the private sector. Over the previous four decades, approximately 10% of the UK's land mass had been sold from public to private ownership. Half of the land that public bodies owned at the beginning of Margaret Thatcher's premiership had been lost to the private sector (Ormerod, 2018c), a process that Brett Christophers has described as the 'new enclosure' (2019: 1).

Accounting tricks have also played a role in balancing the books. One of these has been capital-to-revenue transfers, which allow money that was meant for long-term investment to be used for day-to-day running costs. Such transfers have led to billions of pounds being lost from capital budgets, meaning that trusts were unable to invest in maintenance of estates. The result has been buildings literally falling down (Carey, 2024).[33]

One final way of attempting to navigate financial difficulty has been the use of charitable funding. NHS Charities Together has existed since 2008 but rapidly rose in prominence during the pandemic, when it raised £150 million within a few months (Stewart et al, 2022). In Manchester Universities Foundation Trust in 2023/2024, £1.2m of the £112.1m capital spend was from 'donated and granted assets' In total, £4.7m was raised for the trust charity by 'individuals, companies, community groups, businesses, charitable trusts and foundations' (Manchester University Foundation Trust, 2024: 35). The importance of this source of funds can be understood by looking at what the trust's accounts attribute to it: the purchase of an optical angiography machine in the Eye Hospital, the provision of Safer

Sleep initiatives for infants, the delivery of musical well-being projects at the young person's inpatient mental health unit, and the refurbishment of the paediatric hospital's play area.

COVID-19

When COVID-19 reached the UK in 2020, the UK responded by temporarily increasing the resources available to the NHS. Trusts were told to spend whatever was required to deal with the increased demand on acute hospitals (Calvert and Arbuthnott, 2021). Unfortunately, since capacity had been lost over the previous decade of underfunding, throwing money at the problem in 2020 did not lead to immediately helpful solutions. The resources that had been lost were not ones that could be built up again in such a short period of time: trained staff, appropriate space, hospital beds and relevant equipment. The latter included, famously, personal protective equipment (PPE).[34]

This book will not relitigate the failures of then Prime Minister Boris Johnson and Secretary of State for Health and Social Care Matt Hancock (see Marmot, Allen, Goldblatt, et al, 2020; Thomas, 2020; Calvert and Arbuthnott, 2021; Nazroo and Bécares, 2021; Hyde, 2022). In summary, the crisis that many experts had been warning about for some time finally hit. What had euphemistically been referred to as efficiency gains were now properly recognized as assaults on the 'resilience' of the NHS.[35]

Between 2010 and 2022, the NHS had lost 25,000 beds, meaning it had the second lowest number of beds per 1,000 people in the European Union (which it left in 2020) (Boyle and Chiles, 2022). Before the pandemic, numbers of doctors per capita in the UK were among the lowest in Europe (Eurostat, 2019). Staff vacancies were high, as was turnover.[36] The technology available to staff was severely restricted. For example, in the Organization for Economic Development (OECD), the average amount of imaging machines is 17 MRI machines and 25 CT scanners per million people. The UK had fewer than 10 per million. As one think tank analyst put it, even if policy decisions made during the pandemic were exasperating, 'the problems we faced weren't new. Rather, COVID-19 exposed and exploited structural problems that already existed, only now at a huge scale' (Christopher Thomas, 2022: xiii).

The NHS played a key role in UK political discourse relating to the state's response. From the announcement of the lockdown on 23 March 2020 until 10 May 2020, the government's public health messaging was short and direct: 'Stay home. Protect the NHS. Save lives.' On 31 October 2020, Boris Johnson announced a second national lockdown to prevent 'overrunning the NHS', which would be a 'medical and moral disaster' (Prime Minister's Office, 2020). On 4 January 2021, the Prime Minister addressed the nation again to announce a third lockdown, explaining, 'if action is not taken NHS capacity may be overwhelmed within 21 days' (Prime Minister's Office, 2021). He returned to the original maxim, closing his speech by saying, 'But for now, I am afraid, you must once again stay at home, protect the NHS and save lives.'

Before the vaccine arrived, more people died as a result of COVID-19 than in comparable European countries (Reed, Schlepper and Edwards, 2022). NHS capacity was pushed to the brink, with clinicians enforcing strict triaging decisions that excluded many people from intensive care units that would normally have been accepted, leading to some possibly avoidable deaths (Calvert and Arbuthnott, 2021; Reed, 2024).[37] In the hearings for the COVID-19 public inquiry, Dr Kevin Fong broke down in tears as he spoke of visiting hospitals that were 'bursting at the seams'. Dr Fong recalled a doctor on one unit telling him it was 'like a terrorist attack every day since it started and we don't know when the attacks are going to stop' (Fong, 2024).

Outside of lockdowns, the NHS still featured heavily in the government's messaging. When a contact-tracing organization was launched, it was named 'NHS Test and Trace' even though many of its functions were outsourced to private companies (Pollock, 2020). Similarly, testing centres were branded with the NHS kitemark but run by a variety of outsourced companies (Garside and Neate, 2020; National Audit Office, 2020b).

Ultimately, the vaccine was rolled out from 2021 onwards, making use of the NHS's vast systemic footprint and clinical expertise (Timmins and Baird, 2022), beginning the path towards what we now consider normality.

Tracking healthcare outcomes

Researchers' findings on the impacts of austerity have varied, but have consistently found that it correlated with hundreds of thousands of excess deaths, even before the COVID-19 pandemic (Watkins et al, 2017; Walsh et al, 2022; Berman and Hovland, 2024). Improvements in life expectancy have stalled and inequalities in health have widened (Marmot, Allen, Boyce, et al, 2020). However, the impacts of welfare retrenchment on health were only partially caused by changes in health*care*. Restrictions to welfare payments, housing and social care, as well as public sector pay suppression, have all been relevant. Perhaps moreso. But this is a book about the NHS, so that will be my focus.

One of the stated aims of integration and the purported radical upgrade in community services was to reduce demand for hospital care. The Royal College of Emergency Medicine was skeptical that such an objective could be realized (Royal College of Emergency Medicine, 2017). Their skepticism was well placed. Areas that pioneered integrated care did not see decreases in demand for hospital care, although the increases in those areas were slightly slower than in other areas (Keeble et al, 2019). Emergency admissions in areas with integrated care continued to rise dramatically, and people felt less supported by, and less able to see their general practitioner (Scobie, 2019). Specifically in Greater Manchester, the amount of people waiting over four hours in emergency departments and the amount of time people spent in acute hospital beds remained stubbornly high (Dunhill, 2018; 2020).

COVID-19 then led to a drastic reduction in admissions, as people were advised to steer clear of hospitals to allow them to focus on pandemic admissions. The reduction in admissions persisted beyond the end of the pandemic. However, waiting times continued to rise, partly due to delayed discharges as a result of the collapsing social care system.[38]

Privatization: the buy-out

The self-pay market has grown dramatically in response to increasing waiting times, particularly for outpatient appointments and elective procedures. Waiting lists are at record levels, with 7.6 million awaiting treatment in September 2024.[39] When all forms of care are included, around one fifth of the population report that they are awaiting NHS care, with the most deprived groups reporting the longest waits (Fisher and Taylor, 2024). Employers have also recognized the impact of waiting lists on employees. Therefore employee health insurance has become more common as businesses attempt to get their human capital back to work as quickly as possible.

Before the pandemic, private sector companies openly stated their predictions that restricted NHS budgets would lead to increased use of private healthcare. For example, private healthcare provider Spire published documents in 2018 predicting more NHS e-referrals to private healthcare firms, as well as growth in the market for self-pay healthcare in response to NHS cuts (Investegate, 2019). This analysis of the UK healthcare market was supported by investment bank JP Morgan which noted in 2017 that 'continued structural pressure on the NHS … is likely to lead to more outsourcing to the private sector. If not, we still believe the private sector will benefit as individuals are increasingly forced to dip into their own pockets to fund their care' (quoted by Rowland, 2022: 8). Unlike the NHS's crumbling buildings starved of investment, there was significant investment in private infrastructure.[40]

Spire and JP Morgan were right. The numbers resorting to privately funding their own care (or paying through their employer's health insurance) have risen steadily to reach record heights (Hughes, 2024).[41]

Chris Thomas, think tank researcher and author of a recent book on how to improve the NHS and UK health (2022), somewhat frustratedly contrasts the growth of the self-pay market with that of outsourcing. He calls the first the 'buy-out' and the latter the 'sell-off'.[42]

Privatization: the sell-off

Scholars have found the relationship between restricted funds and privatization difficult to pin down. Krachler and Greer (2015) argue that decreased state funding for healthcare in other countries, such as Germany, has led to increased privatization. In 2015, they wondered why the same had not happened in the UK. They argued that campaigners' efforts to keep health 'highly politicized' (Krachler and Greer, 2015: 222) had contributed to the failure of private companies to gain a foothold in the UK. Seaton's (2023) history agrees with their thesis, as will this book, to some degree. However, the sell-off actually *has* advanced since they posed the puzzle. That is, it is becoming clearer that there is less of a puzzle to solve.

Before the pandemic, the government's own figures stated that it spends approximately 7% on the private sector (The King's Fund, 2019) and that this figure had remained fairly consistent over the past few years. But these figures did not include payments to the voluntary sector, nor did they include payments to GPs and NHS dentists, which have always operated as independent contractors (Rowland, 2019). When including all English health spending that goes to organizations that are not NHS trusts or other statutory bodies, the figure rose to 22% of total expenditure (Buckingham and Dayan, 2019), with the numbers gradually increasing over the years. The new Labour government is keen to publicize increasing usage of the private sector, announcing '6.15 million tests and operations for NHS patients were delivered by independent healthcare providers over the past year – almost 500,000 more than last year … Using spare capacity in the private sector is central to the government's goal' (Department of Health and Social Care and Streeting, 2025).[43]

Ancillary services that are outsourced within a trust are not included in the figures outlined above. This outsourcing is staring you in the face when you walk into any NHS hospital. In 2025, cleaners, maintenance workers, security staff, catering staff and porters are all likely to employed by one of the Big Four contractors listed above.[44] Chapter 3 follows one example of a group of NHS workers campaigning not to be outsourced, in that case to a company wholly owned by the NHS trust, rather than one of the Big Four.

More recent (and complete) figures do highlight increasing NHS spending on private companies, with 7.5% of planned NHS admissions being provided by the private sector in 2022/2023, an increase of 30% that year (Dayan, Gainsbury and Bagri, 2024).[45] The private sector now regularly reports treating record numbers of NHS patients each quarter (Independent Healthcare Providers Network, 2025). Although outsourcing of NHS work has increased everywhere, it has not done so equally. In some places, up to 20% of elective work is undertaken in private hospitals (Goodair, Bach-Mortensen and Reeves, 2024).[46]

The changes to the structure of the NHS that have taken place since my fieldwork have opened up further opportunities for outsourcing. In 2022, the UK parliament passed the Health and Care Act. This legislation formalized the role of integrated care systems (ICSs), which were what followed after the STPs and ACOs mentioned earlier, which will be discussed at greater length in Chapter 3.[47] ICSs are bigger than the previous commissioning bodies, CCGs. In Greater Manchester, ten CCGs have been replaced by one ICS. In South West England, a company owned by private equity has taken advantage of this larger footprint to secure the contract for provision of all community-based care in one ICP, worth £1.3bn over nine years (Talora, 2024).

In July 2024, Labour returned to power with a landslide victory in the general election. The new government commissioned an investigation by Lord Darzi (Darzi, 2024), announced a moderate increase to funding, committed to addressing the growing waiting lists, launched a public consultation and abolished NHS England. In 2025, it launched the 10 Year Plan (Department of Health and Social Care, 2025).[48] However, it has been observed that the amount of money allocated to the NHS will be swallowed by inflation and salary increases for existing workers (McLellan, 2024). Therefore, trusts will actually experience real terms cuts. Furthermore, Prime Minister Keir Starmer and Secretary of State for Health and Social Care Wes Streeting[49] have bullishly signalled a willingness to use the private sector, even bringing class discourse into their reasoning, with Streeting stating that he was willing to ignore the 'howls of outrage' from 'middle-class Lefties' who opposed the use of the private sector (Penna, 2024).[50] Again, we see the narrative of a declining NHS, but here used against the activists with whom I did fieldwork.

Conclusion

This chapter has given a simple timeline outlining a history of the policy changes that have led to cuts and privatization in the NHS. Although we have seen glimpses of other narratives, such as those that point towards welfare nationalism, in most part I have constructed a narrative that, since the neoliberal period ushered in by Thatcher, successive governments have reduced the real-terms funding of the NHS and attempted to open it up to the market. I focused on negative healthcare outcomes that have occurred recently. I chose these based on the kinds of outcomes that I heard activists worrying about and using in their discourse. In their arguments, poor outcomes have occurred as a result of cuts and privatization. The basic through-line of the chapter narrative has been that, just as Galen pointed out, activists continue to defend something that is becoming less defensible.

What did Galen mean? As the next chapters will elaborate, what activists imagined the NHS to be – and what they aspired and hoped that the NHS could be – was being eroded. Activists believed the NHS was becoming less *good*. Delving into what they meant when they talked about the NHS will help us to understand their constructions of the good, and their undertakings – personal, relational, collective and institutional – to realize that good. Historians such as Bivins (2015) and Crane (2019), who have documented the NHS both as a site in which racism is enacted and also opposed, provide a potential answer to Galen's question; defence might be through a counter-mobilization of the icon, a contestation of its meaning. This book tracks the ways in which he and other activists answered their question in practice. Rather than accept a meaning of the NHS as given, such as a racist, exclusionary one that they considered indefensible, they constructed their own meaning. They used and built on particular narratives with a particular interpretation of the NHS, mobilizing its iconicity in particular ways to particular ends with particular social and material consequences.

3

Fears of Privatization

On 1 March 2019, Ronny, a member of the Socialist Health Association tweeted, 'The conspiracy theorists who complained that the NHS internal market was introducing privatization are now shouting that abolishing it will introduce privatization.' A journalist from *Health Service Journal* (HSJ) – a periodical that is widely read and well respected by NHS managers – replied sarcastically, 'Everything is privatising the NHS'.

Ronny and the HSJ journalist were mocking activists by describing them as conspiracy theorists. It was an accusation activists were used to, and which they refuted. Yet the observation that 'Everything is privatising the NHS' spoke to a truth I had noticed during fieldwork. Most of the activists I spent time with in Keep Our NHS Public (KONP), Greater Manchester KONP and Dunning KONP evaluated all new announcements, policies and reforms to work out if and how they could lead to privatization, and contested them on that basis. Moreover, the question of *whether* a particular reform could lead to privatization was often elided, facilitating a progression straight to the more vexed question of *how* it would. It was this elision that Ronny was pointing out.[1]

This chapter explores how activists' fears of privatization shaped their actions. The chapter has three aims: first, I explore the moral fact of the wrongness of privatization.[2] In interviews, when I asked activists the direct question of what made privatization wrong, they usually replied that privatization led to worse healthcare. Second, I make sense of the relationship between this consequentialist argument and that of Chapter 1, which considered the NHS as an example of socialism. I draw on Keane (2010) to make the case that outcomes-based arguments were explicit surface arguments chosen for being persuasive. But other implicit rationales also emerged through examination of all of the ethnographic material. Thick description of activists' narratives regarding their memories of struggles against privatization – protecting the idea of an NHS that provided care for all – reveals how we might understand these consequentialist arguments as contemporary salvos in an ethico-political battle with a long history. The current phase continues to be one in which certain forms of argumentation hold more currency than others: namely, 'what matters is what works'. But activists' interpretation of what worked depended on a different ethical unit of interest, derived from the NHS value of universality. For activists, what mattered was what worked for the whole population, rather than particular individuals.

Third, I consider the puzzle that so enervated Ronny and the HSJ journalist. Why do NHS activists interpret every attempt at reforming the NHS as a step towards privatization? Their arguments were focused on future dangers, but heavily influenced by their understandings of the past, in which the NHS symbolized the state's capacity to resist the power of private capital. I develop an argument that considers their fear as a critique of the vulnerability of the contemporary state in the face of global capital. After Chapter 1, this chapter provides another perspective on the temporality of NHS activists.[3] I demonstrate how, in their temporality, they considered that the future was to be feared, but that through collective struggle, they could temper the worst aspects of privatization.

However, reading their critique as justifiable misses an important point. Their understanding of the NHS as *good* – morally, materially, practically – contributed to nonchalance regarding the pre-existing structure of the NHS. In the final section I examine the privatization that has taken place in general practice. I argue that activists' fearful engagement with change blunted cold analysis of the inherited institutional deposits from which their material understanding of the good was formed. The temporality of fear regarding the future was based on a morally foundational view of what was to be protected that diverted attention from inherent dangers within the original organization of the NHS. I return to Keane's work in the anthropology of ethics to demonstrate that an artificial separation of material life and the ideal or internal ethical judgement of it cannot be sustained. The material institution of the NHS became intertwined with the moral understanding of what it meant to be good, thus occluding views of where material reality did not align with aspirations.

What did activists mean by 'privatization'?

Healthcare privatization is defined by Krachler and Greer as 'a change in ownership in which non-state actors become increasingly involved in provision, usually through a transfer of assets (e.g. the sale of a hospital) or an increase in work contracted out' (2015: 216). This is a definition that most of the activists I worked with would accept, although many would add that it is not just providers of care that can be privatized. The organizations that commission care can also be privatized, an important point for this chapter, which focuses on ACOs, organizations involved both in commissioning and providing services.[4]

Occasionally, managers and politicians worked with narrower understandings of what constituted privatization. They argued that a service contracted out to a private company would not constitute privatization if the NHS – the state – was footing the bill. For them, privatization meant people *paying* specifically for healthcare rather than receiving it free-at-the-point-of-use.[5]

Managers who followed the narrower definition of privatization often cited General Practitioners (GPs) as an example of independent contractors who should not be considered as privatized entities, since they provided NHS services, free to patients, almost exclusively. The case of GPs was a moot one among Keep Our NHS Public (KONP) members. Managers and politicians tended to consider activists' silence on GPs – even as they criticized other independent sector organizations – as evidence of either ignorance or inconsistency.

The activists that I spoke to were not ignorant of the GP contractor model, nor were they entirely comfortable with it. But as it was a pre-existing model that had not changed recently,[6] it was not at the forefront of their attention. They did not consider their opposition to new privatization as inconsistent with an awareness of GPs' semi-independence. The focus of activists' critical attention on programmes of change rather than pre-existing structures is something that I will return to in the final sections of the chapter. I will argue that the temporality of fear was inherently linked to the conceptualization of the NHS as a moral example.

The activists I spent time with would also disagree with Krachler and Greer's definition's focus on the non-state ownership of assets. Activists were keenly aware that state bodies employed staff on different terms and conditions to companies, and were subject to different kinds of regulation and taxation, even if the companies were owned by state bodies. During my fieldwork, some NHS trusts sought to take advantage of these differences, for example through transferring staff to newly formed subsidiary companies that remained wholly owned by the trust. Assets did not transfer into the ownership of particular individuals. But activists still understood such actions as privatization and contested them as such, as in the case of Wigan, discussed in this chapter.

Accountable Care Organizations as a case example of the fear of privatization

Background on ACOs

NHS England announced in March 2017 that all Sustainability and Transformation Plans (STPs, the geographical footprints envisaged as a way of enacting the 5 Year Forward View) were to eventually evolve into ACOs.[7] The ACO would be the single organization that a Clinical Commissioning

Group (CCG) could commission to provide all health and social care in an integrated manner.

The term, ACO, originates in the US, where it forms a part of the Kaiser Permanente model of 'managed care' and was used in the Affordable Care Act. Like Health Maintenance Organizations, ACOs are paid by insurers to provide comprehensive medical care for people who are insured. Insurers pay a block amount per patient, and providers decide what care they include for the block price, that is, what they consider as 'comprehensive'. Theoretically, the contractual mechanism allows insurers to hold ACOs 'accountable' for the services provided.

Immediately after the announcement of draft ACO contracts in August 2017, think tanks began to publish articles on implications for the NHS. Activists also began to discuss implications. In November 2017, a group of doctors, academics and health campaigners calling themselves #JR4NHS[8] announced that they were seeking a judicial review of the lawfulness of ACOs. Stephen Hawking's involvement as one of the litigants helped to create a national buzz around the case. None of the people I worked with in Greater Manchester were part of #JR4NHS, but they all followed the case closely, and Dunning KONP made regular contributions to its crowdfund. The judicial review affected the local context in that while it was ongoing, plans for anything that resembled an ACO were put on hold.

Ultimately, the judicial review failed to uphold that ACOs were illegal. However, the result of the wide reporting of the case, as well as a concurrent investigation of ACOs by the Parliamentary Select Committee on Health and Social Care (Health and Social Care Committee, 2018), was a change of direction from NHS England. They decided to encourage organizations to move towards ICPs (integrated care partnerships) rather than ACOs. Essentially, ICPs were very similar but had been rebranded so as not to sound American (Ham, 2018) (Manchester actually ended up having an *LCO*, rather than an ACO).[9]

Ultimately, ACOs never came into existence. They were replaced by Integrated Care Systems, discussed in *The Internal Market* section of Chapter 2. At the time of my fieldwork, ACOs were still a live issue. I will use activists' engagement with ACOs to demonstrate how they looked out for *and found* pathways to privatization in all proposed reforms.

Activist engagement with ACOs

In the first few months of my fieldwork, it was far from clear what ACOs were or what they would do. Activists were alarmed at their American origins. Much of the literature published by activist organizations took the American link as evidence that the chief executive of NHS England, Simon Stevens – already considered a suspicious character because he used to work for United Health – was attempting to 'Americanize the NHS'. Having made the link to the US healthcare system, the dangers of ACOs in England were easy to identify, by simply observing what had already gone wrong in the US.

I first saw the following list of dangers in an email newsletter sent by the National Health Action Party, a political party set up in 2012 in response to the Health and Social Care Act. The same list was re-used in literature published by the activist organizations with whom I worked, including Health Campaigns Together (HCT) and Dunning KONP.

1. ACOs will be given the money for your care as an insurance premium, and will pay out only for certain treatments – like an insurance company.
2. ACOs will in many cases be handed over to actual insurance companies and other private firms.
3. ACOs will be able to decide what care is free and what they can charge patients for.
4. ACOs will be paid more if they 'save' money (e.g. spend less money on front-line services).
5. ACOs will be subject to commercial rules and will hide behind the veil of 'corporate confidentiality'.
6. ACOs are not recognized in any Act of Parliament and as such have no legal basis.

A Dunning KONP leaflet in February 2018 repeated the same list and added one more point:

7. ACOs will mark the end of the NHS as a comprehensive health service that provides healthcare to us all, based on our clinical needs.

Points 1 and 2 essentially say that ACOs are a step towards private insurance, and thus towards privatized healthcare. (These points build on the criticism of STPs that it broke the NHS into bite-size chunks that were more appetizing to private healthcare companies looking to invest in UK healthcare.) Points 3–5 illustrate some of the problems with the private insurance model.[10] These points echo what activists told me in interviews when I asked them what was wrong with privatization in general.

Points 3–5 and my informants' answers to the question of what was wrong with privatization can be summarized as saying that private healthcare provides care that is worse for patients because it is driven by a profit incentive rather than some other, more benign motive. Thus the profit motive – at least in healthcare – is *wrong* insofar as it leads to worse healthcare, at least at a population level. Some people may be able to afford to pay more for better healthcare, thus leading to inequality of access to healthcare.

I concentrate on two observations in this chapter. First, if worse care is the premise upon which the ethical objection to private healthcare is based, then private healthcare can only be understood as wrong if you suppose that the ethical unit of interest is the whole population. This is because if the ethical unit of interest is the whole population, then the possibility that private healthcare *might* provide better healthcare for an individual becomes irrelevant. I will return to the importance of this ethical unit of interest when I consider the various ways arguments were mobilized that were based on a rubric of 'what matters is what works'.

Second, points 1–7 all use the future tense in the indicative mood. They are not presented as conjecture or possibility. They are predictions. They are engagements with the morality of the *present* through a consideration of *future* consequences, presented as facts rather than possibilities. In sum, privatization is wrong, and ACOs are wrong because they move us closer to privatization. Furthermore, we can locate what activists felt to be right by considering the opposite of the wrong, that is, publicly owned bodies, or the NHS as activists imagined it to be at some point in the past. Particular memories of the past contribute to a sense of what is right, and what is potentially to be lost, thus affording a moral apparatus to apprehend the present.

In the next section, I focus on a conference organized to discuss ACOs, in which activists further revealed how their fears of privatization shaped their understandings of ACOs.

SHA conference on ACOs

On 25 November 2017, I attended a conference organized by Ronny for the Socialist Health Association (SHA). He had invited a number of managers, activists and academics to give talks based on their own research or experience of ACOs. When the conference started, several speakers were critical of ACOs, making links with American healthcare similar to those listed above. Several were more positive. While only one of the critics came from an NHS management background, all of the people speaking more positively were current or recent NHS managers. I concentrate on the talk given by John Lister,[11] a London campaigner well known in NHS activism for *London Health Emergency*, an anti-cuts, anti-privatization periodical that he was a founding editor of in the 1980s. At the time of the conference, in 2017, he was still active, as co-chair of KONP and editor of *Health Campaigns Together*. In his own words, he had 'been campaigning against privatization for 33 years, or since God wore shorts, basically'.

In his talk, he gave a potted history of the NHS since Thatcher. In his narrative, every government from the 1980s onwards, including New Labour, had contributed to a 'constant cranking up of marketization'. He included some figures, for example, that the total NHS spend on private providers of care was £200m under Thatcher. The NHS was now spending £800m just on private mental health beds.[12] He recognized that there had been a change of tone in NHS policy under Simon Stevens. He welcomed some of the discourse around STPs, particularly around better care, closer to people's homes, but heavily criticized the lack of democratic input into or credible financial scrutiny of their plans.

When he got to ACOs, his critique was not that they would lead to privatization. It was that:

1. people had already lost trust with STPs due to the lack of democratic input, and were unlikely to trust anything that had a name taken from the American model;
2. total NHS funding was woefully inadequate;
3. the social care system was already privatized and dysfunctional.

He approved of the concept of ACOs as 'the basis for a fully integrated, publicly planned and provided system'. But the problem was that the factors listed above would get in the way of them working. Regarding the danger of privatization, he simply said, 'the Americans aren't coming. Why would they? Insurers make all the money. Providers take all the risk.'

The discussion following his talk was heated; attendees took issue with his understandings of the dangers. Lemmy, an NHS administrator and KONP member from Liverpool, contended that 'the privatization agenda has not been ditched. It has been disguised.' He added, 'the Americans *are* coming' and pointed to the presence of Centene, an American healthcare provider, in Nottingham. Lister replied that Centene were only operating a £2.5 million contract for non-clinical services, 'a drop in the ocean' out of the NHS budget. And the lack of funds was the most urgent danger to deal with. Lemmy added that it might be a small contract, but it was just them 'dipping their toe in the water. If it works, the rest will come behind them.' Several members of Dunning KONP nodded when Lemmy said this.

The discussions continued in this vein. Some people highlighted the dangers of ACOs, namely privatization. Others minimized such dangers. For both groups, the undesirability of privatized healthcare was not in question. By the end of the conference, most of the attendees had not decided that ACOs definitely would or would not lead to privatization. The point I wish to illustrate is that everyone was avidly looking for the ways in which ACOs *could* lead to privatization. Even Lister was on the lookout for dangers, although he did not see privatization as *the most immediate* threat. Towards the end of the conference, he qualified his argument, suggesting that American companies were not investing as much money in the UK as they were in, for example, Brazil and Chile, but that we should be wary of British companies, such as Virgin. In summary, there was some disagreement over whether ACOs *would* lead to privatization, but the consensus was that a danger existed that ACOs *could* be privatized. In the next sections, I follow how the 'could' hardened into 'would'.

ACOs and tendering

The conference provided a microcosm for debates that were taking place among activists nationally.[13] Dunning KONP followed local developments closely, attending council and Clinical Commissioning Group (CCG) meetings and discussing the plans for eventual evolution into an ACO. About halfway through my fieldwork, Danny, a member of Dunning KONP as well as a councillor, reported to the group that the council had decided that they would not progress to an ACO, and would instead function as a 'loose alliance'. Dunning KONP welcomed this news but remained vigilant. Vigilant for what? One of their concerns throughout had been that ACOs could be privatized. When assured by councillors and managers that they were working under plans for the local NHS to be run by a partnership between the council and the CCG – that is, by collaboration between state bodies – they were not reassured. Activists argued that even if they took managers' and politicians' arguments in good faith, their promises only lasted as long as they were in post, or as long as the length of one contract. Unless the Health and Social Care Act (the Act) was revoked, the legislation remained in place that forced any new contract to be put out to tender again.

The same fear applied to central Manchester, where I was told by several people that the managers and politicians involved in setting up the LCO on its first ten-year contract had made efforts to ensure that Virgin would not be able to win the contract. Ronny, who sat as a lay member of the public on the Manchester Health and Care Commissioning (MHCC) Patient and Public Advisory Group (PPAG), and thus had some input into the LCO contract, told me it was 'fixed' so that MHCC would win the contract, that is, so that the state would retain control and ownership.[14] Even so, at the end of the ten-year contract, unless legislation had changed, it would be put out to tender again, with different managers and politicians in place who may be less wary of privatization.

When managers and politicians felt they had taken steps to avoid privatization, and to demonstrate to activists that they had done so, activists continued to search for *and find* ways that the proposed reorganizations could still lead to privatization, even if that possibility was ten years away. Activists' engagement with ACOs has illuminated the ever-present fear of privatization and the search prompted by this fear. Next I explain the source of this fear by discussing some of the predictions made by NHS activists.

Memories of struggles against privatization

As discussed in Chapter 1, Dunning KONP was set up in response to the Health and Social Care Act. However, my friends in other parts of Greater Manchester had been campaigning against cuts and privatization for decades. They viewed the Act not as a rupture, but as just another event in a long history of increasing private involvement in the NHS in particular, and in state welfare services in general. That history, as they saw it, had begun with Thatcher and continued under Blair and Brown.

Catherine, Ruth, Olga and Nancy, all long-term members of Greater Manchester KONP, told me of the various struggles they had been involved in, many before they had joined KONP. All of them had worked in the NHS and been active in their unions. Catherine and Ruth were now retired from their roles in public health. Olga still worked as a mental health nurse. Nancy still worked in healthcare administration, but reorganizations following the Act had meant that she was now employed by local government rather than the NHS.

Unlike Dunning KONP members, Greater Manchester KONP members were able to give a list of examples of previous moves they had opposed, and how their activism had slowed privatization down. For example, when foundation trusts were announced, activists opposed them on the basis that the newly found independence of the organizations meant: (a) that whole trusts could be privatized in the future; and (b) trusts would have more freedom to outsource services to private companies.[15] Importantly, their organizing was based not just on laying out the possible paths to privatization, but on arguing that those paths *would* be followed, that is, that trusts would increase their outsourcing. Catherine lamented the failure of their campaigning to stop the change in policy from coming into place, but pointed to the fact that only one trust in the country had in fact been privatized.[16] Outsourcing of specific services had continued to increase, but Catherine argued that it would have been even greater had there been less campaigning in the first place.[17]

Most Greater Manchester KONP members' previous struggles had been as members of their respective unions, and many of their stories overlapped, including a strike by nurses, in response to Olga's dismissal by an NHS trust in 2007.[18] Olga's alleged misdemeanour had been bringing the trust into disrepute by writing an article that criticized a third sector organization that the trust considered a partner. Olga told me that the article did not name specific organizations, but did say that outsourcing services to third sector organizations was worse for staff as they were no longer protected by NHS terms and conditions, and worse for patients as they could be managed by less qualified or unqualified staff.

When the trust dismissed her, the union launched a dispute in which they argued that the real reason for Olga's dismissal was her criticism of the cuts being made at the time by the trust. Olga had predicted that cuts would in themselves worsen the provision of care, but also that cuts would lead to further privatization, that privatization would lead to worse services, and that worse services would lead to bad outcomes for patients. Through the union, she had attempted to galvanize the workforce into objecting to the cuts on the basis that they would lead to privatization.

Other clinicians that I spoke to about the strike remembered it as a euphoric time, despite the ultimately negative result. Olga never got her job back. When I asked them to reflect on the negative result, they returned the same answer: it would have been worse if we had not protested. The service Olga was working in was not cut (at the time), which they all considered as evidence of the partial success of the dispute. However, other services were cut, and other services were outsourced. Olga, Catherine, Nancy and Ruth all argued that *more* services would have been cut and/or privatized if they had not objected, and the strike was one manifestation of these objections.

The salience of their belief that their actions had stopped or slowed privatization can be illustrated by considering a strike that occurred during my fieldwork. In early 2018, Wrightington, Wigan and Leigh NHS Foundation Trust announced plans to outsource many of its non-clinical staff to a wholly owned subsidiary company. The staff objected, since this would mean no longer being NHS staff, with nationally agreed terms and conditions, negotiated through collective bargaining. Their union, Unison, announced a strike. Greater Manchester KONP and Dunning KONP agreed to support the industrial action. Along with Catherine, Ruth, Olga, Lily and Leroy, I attended a picket in May 2018. Following the strike (as well as closed-door discussions between the trust, the council, MPs and the Mayor), the trust backed down and shelved the plans. The industrial action had stopped the contracting out to a private company (in this case one wholly owned by the trust).

One further detail regarding this strike is pertinent. I had interviewed a senior manager at the trust in October 2017, several months before any of us knew of the looming outsourcing. During the interview, he had described part of his role as reducing the anxieties and fears of staff, especially when large reforms were underway. He found that NHS activists were often unhelpful in this regard, since they came up with wild 'conspiracy theories' that filtered through to staff. He was referring to activists' fears of cuts and privatization, which he told me were unrealistic. A few months later, the trust attempted to contract out many of its staff. He had played a major role in realizing the thing that he had told me was unrealistic.

Owing to research confidentiality, I never told Greater Manchester KONP or Dunning KONP members about this interview, even when standing on the picket outside Wigan Hospital. If I had done so, I am fairly sure they would have considered it in the same way they considered the reassurances of managers and politicians that ACOs would remain under public ownership. They would have been suspicious. At best, they would have suspected naivety. At worst, dissembling. Either way, they would not have been reassured that a manager telling them they did not need to worry about privatization really meant that they had nothing to worry about.

Conservative thinking

Activists' also explained their fears through reference to the discourse of politicians, especially Tories. They often mentioned previous publications written by Tory politicians, including Oliver Letwin and John Redwood's *Britain's Biggest Enterprise – Ideas for Radical Reform of the NHS* (1988) and Jeremy Hunt's contribution to *Direct Democracy: An Agenda for a New Model Party* (Direct Democracy, 2005).[19] Since Hunt was Secretary of State for Health for most of my fieldwork, activists mentioned the latter publication much more often. However, they did occasionally mention the former as well, connecting the dots to argue that Letwin and Redwood's work shows that the Tories have always wanted to privatize the NHS. Hunt's work showed that they still did. When I suggested to Dunning KONP that Hunt had made more recent statements that the Tories had no intention to privatize the NHS, Iris replied, 'Well, he would say that, wouldn't he?' Her implication was clear: the Tories still wanted to privatize parts or all of the NHS. If he stated otherwise, he was not being entirely truthful.[20]

Greater Manchester KONP members, including Catherine, Ruth, Olga and Nancy, did not exempt Labour politicians from neoliberal influence or participation in the 'revolving door' between politics and high-paid consultancy roles in the private sector. Their narratives of resisting privatization included memories between 1997 and 2010, before the Tory Party returned to power. The IEA's influence on the Tory Party was just the most recent chapter of a longer history in their eyes.[21]

When I attended a fringe event at the Tory party conference in October 2017, I myself witnessed a discrepancy between what Tory politicians said to the wider public and what they said behind closed doors. Although it was open to anyone, the audience at the event was restricted to mostly Tories since it was not widely publicized and one had to sign up to attend. I had come across it by accident while scanning the Tory party conference's website.

In this particular audience, Stephen Dorrell, then chair of the NHS Confederation,[22] formerly Tory Secretary of State for Health, stood up from the floor and suggested that the state should not be the preferred provider of any kind of public service. He referred to a political consensus that he attributed to Tony Blair, of 'what matters is what works', meaning that if a budgetary decision maker found that a private company could provide a service, then he/she should not balk at the prospect of privatization. Philip

Dunne, then Minister of State for Health, agreed and said there was scope for more privatization. David Hare, chief executive of the NHS Partners Network (which represents independent and private sector organizations that provide NHS services), also agreed, saying that the problem with reducing the provision of private healthcare through the NHS is that it would mean that only those who could afford private healthcare would buy private healthcare.

The only voice of disagreement came from the chief executive of the NHS Confederation, Niall Dickson. His disagreement was not with the substance of what Dorrell, Dunne and Hare had said. Instead he worried about transparency. He noted that there was a difference between what people were saying in the room and what the same people were saying to the wider public. He argued that if the politicians and managers wanted more independent sector involvement in the provision of NHS services then they should say so publicly. But this disparity between public pronouncements and ulterior motives was no surprise to members of Dunning KONP and Greater Manchester KONP. When I reported back to them, they rolled their eyes and assured me that they already knew what the Tories were up to. They did not need *further* evidence that people in power had an intention to privatize. The next – more urgent – task was to figure out how they were going to go about doing so and oppose their moves.

Privatization is wrong

In my interviews with activists, I often asked directly, 'What is wrong with privatization?' The most common answer was that the private sector generally provided worse care. Points 3–5 on the ACO leaflet provide an example of the basic structure of the argument: the profit motive incentivizes cost-cutting, which leads to worse care.[23]

Often, activists provided me with concrete examples of where privatization had led to a deterioration in outcomes. For example, they referred to Circle's takeover of an already-existing NHS hospital in Cambridgeshire in 2012.[24] As described in Chapter 1, Leroy often compared publicly owned healthcare in the UK to private healthcare in the US. Leroy mentioned the US most times that I saw him, and others often referred to it as well, hence the anxiety at the ACO conference regarding whether the 'Americans are coming'. Occasionally, activists referred to their own negative experiences of private healthcare, in the UK or the US.

The moral argument I have described is a consequentialist, utilitarian one: privatization leads to worse care and therefore worse health *for more people*. Although the description of private healthcare as 'profit driven' was tinged with disapproval of the profit motive itself, that disapproval was hitched to this consequentialist argument, rather than one grounded in political economy. Rather than anything approaching Marx's allusions to capitalists as vampires feasting on the value extracted from workers, whose freedom and flourishing they had curtailed under conditions of wage slavery, activists much more often referred more mildly to the naivety or dishonesty of local state actors. The possibility that unequal relations between capitalists and workers might be consolidated by healthcare privatization, engendering further inequality, was not mentioned.[25]

However, at times, snippets of other rationales for opposing privatization have revealed themselves in this chapter. John Lister spoke of democratic input and public control. The healthcare staff engaged in industrial action in Wigan were worried regarding the terms of their employment. The article for which Olga suffered disciplinary action spoke not just of worse care for patients, but also worse conditions for staff. In Lister's discourse, and the two industrial actions, we see fragments of the wider goods that egalitarian arguments are based on, ones that could mesh with the argument of Chapter 1, that the NHS was an example of socialism and was to be protected *as such*.

How can we reconcile the recurring utilitarian arguments with the scraps of other kinds of moral discourse that also surfaced? I consider that the consequentialist focus on patient outcomes was a form of explicit moral reasoning. Webb Keane, an anthropologist of ethics (2010), argues that reasoning may be tacit or explicit. Tacit ethical reasoning generally follows the expectations or obligations set within a particular 'moral system' (2010: 69), such as the habitual brushing of one's teeth that remains unquestioned most of the time. However, since moral systems are not bounded cultural entities, nor are they mechanistic and totalizing, the placement of ethical reasoning within a moral system does not *explain* it. When called upon to explain herself and her actions, a person's reasoning must become explicit. She must give reasons for her actions, either to herself or others. Such explanations respond to the 'surfaces of things' (2010: 68), by which Keane means people's historically and culturally informed perceptions of the people and environment around them,[26] the phenomena rather than the noumena.

For Keane, two issues arise from making tacit reasoning explicit. First, the reasoning changes as it becomes explicit. Second, making it explicit is an intervention in the world and in social relations, exposing the rationale to response and critique. The actor attempts to make their explicit arguments as persuasive as possible. Therefore, looking at the ways in which activists make explicit arguments may reveal a lot not just about their tacit reasoning, but also their perceptions of the whole moral system.

In what ways do the explicit arguments of NHS activists – that privatization is wrong because it leads to worse outcomes for patients – respond to the surfaces of things? How can we make sense of activists settling on consequentialist arguments? When I asked activists about privatization in interviews, I used the language of morality; I asked what was wrong. But the arguments that they were making were ones that they would take into their engagements with the people and organizations that were restructuring healthcare. They were in a political battle in which they were, as Keane (2010) writes, exposing their arguments to response and critique. They were making the moral political. They had to consider what kinds of arguments were most likely to be persuasive with those people and organizations.

The environment in which they took these arguments was one in which the guiding philosophy was Tony Blair's (and Stephen Dorrell's) dictum that 'what matters is what works'. But they turned Dorrell's pragmatism on its head. Whereas at the Tory conference event, Dorrell had used such logic to promote privatization, NHS activists provided empirical evidence, such as the failure of Circle, to ground the opposite argument. If what matters is what works, then there are no grounds for privatization, since it does not work.

I do not intend to argue either that activists or Blair and Dorrell were correct. Rather, the argument of each set of actors would benefit from unpicking, not least on what it means for something to 'work'. In doing so, we get closer to uncovering the tacit reasoning underneath. As chair of the NHS Confederation, it was Dorrell's job to represent the interests of both public and private sector providers of healthcare. What worked for him was informed by what kept the private sector afloat. He could also correctly argue that the private sector was able to provide better care for some individuals than was being provided on the NHS. In this sense, for Dorrell, 'what matters is what works' described a consequentialist argument that was not utilitarian. The greatest happiness for the greatest number was not his aim. Better outcomes for *some* patients was. On the other hand, the evidence put forward by activists spoke of a wider public. They argued that privatization of specific services led to worse care and worse outcomes *overall*.[27]

Although Dorrell, Dunne and Hare may have argued that their concern was also for the whole public, the main function of the statement, 'what matters is what works', is obfuscation. That is, it obscures exactly what it means to 'work', and in whose benefit such work might result. The public, and questions of where the boundaries of the public are or should be, recede from view. As medical anthropologist Ruth Prince (2014: 2) puts it, the 'public' is 'empt[ied] out … as an inclusive terrain', without the question being raised as to whose interests are being served or denied. Although the statement is presented as neutral and apolitical, it is in fact depoliticizing (Shore and Wright, 1997; 2011). Thus we cannot really know exactly who Dorrell had in mind as the key unit of concern: an individual citizen, the whole population, or the private companies it was his job to represent. However, we can follow the sociological method of evaluating who benefits from such discourse: private health companies and (possibly) the individuals able to afford healthcare from such companies.[28]

The outcomes of interest to Dorrell were at the level of the individual, where it was *possible* that a private entity may provide better care. But the outcomes of interest to NHS activists were for the whole population. They considered the consequences for the whole *society* and found privatization wanting. Moreover, in their political arguments, they made the moral consequences of privatization explicit. Whereas Dorrell's use of pragmatic rhetoric obscured *who* might benefit from privatization, activists exposed how the ethical unit that mattered to them – the whole population – would not benefit. If a reform to the NHS – in this case, privatization, even the privatization of one small part of the NHS – will not improve care for *all*, then it cannot be considered right or good. The NHS, as activists remembered and imagined it, a state-funded public institution, must be protected from the wrongs of privatization.

The ethics of solidarity

It could be argued that I have conflated ethics and politics, and that some of the objections to privatization were not ethical at all. For example, it would be reasonable to assume that the staff engaging in the industrial dispute in Wigan were motivated by immediate self-interest. I believe they probably were. Posing the question of self-interest raises two further questions: Does the existence of a self-interest argument preclude the existence of a moral argument? Did people object to privatization simply because it was an undesirable consequence for a particular group of people, or was it morally wrong? One final question to reconcile these two questions: How might it be possible to argue that both were true: that privatization was wrong *because* it was not in the interests of a specific group of public sector workers?

Let us consider the two strikes. First, Greater Manchester KONP and Dunning KONP members joined a picket in Wigan. I attended with a group of people that were not employees of Wrightington, Wigan and Leigh NHS Foundation Trust, and so were not directly affected by the proposed outsourcing. Explicitly, they argued that their motivation for participating in the protest was that privatization was wrong. One could only argue that their interests were threatened if it could be shown that the outsourcing of staff in Wigan in some way harmed them. Such an argument would align with what social movements scholars (Levi and Olsen, 2000; Silver, 2003) describe as membership of a community of interests, that is, a group of people who feel that they have an identity of interests. If members of Greater Manchester KONP and Dunning KONP felt that their interests were harmed by a change in the terms and conditions of employment of staff in Wigan, they must all consider themselves members of a single community of interests.

The relationship between people in this community of interests is one of solidarity, which Levi and Olsen (2000: 313) describe thus:

> Solidarity depends on a complex and long-term understanding of interests in which members of one union come to believe in the link between their situation and that of others. 'An injury to one is an injury to all,' the slogan of the International Longshore and Warehouse Union (ILWU), epitomizes such a belief. But how is that 'one' defined?

The question of how the community of interest is defined is central to a consideration of how to answer the question of 'what works'. What works *for whom*? The universality of the NHS was central to the moral system that underpinned Dunning KONP and Greater Manchester KONP members' arguments. The health service was universal insofar as it provided care for everyone.[29] Therefore, worse health outcomes in Wigan ought to be rejected by everyone in the UK.

But what about worse terms and conditions for staff in Wigan? The conscious unification of different communities of interest was seen most clearly in Olga's description of what was wrong with outsourcing in 2007: it would lead to worse working conditions for staff,[30] and *therefore* worse care for patients. That is, the question of what works was realigned to focus on what works for staff, because what works for staff influences what works for patients at a macro level. This realigned focus provided an interests-based motive to engage in solidaristic action. Returning to the Wigan strike, members of Greater Manchester KONP and Dunning KONP were willing to protest for the protection of the interests of others, even when their own were not in direct question. But I have demonstrated that consideration of the tacit moral system of NHS activism allowed for an understanding that their interests were indirectly threatened by the outsourcing of staff in Wigan. Their solidarity contributed to the success of the staff in overturning the initial move to outsourcing. Their moral objection had political consequences.

To summarize, I have argued that explications of the wrongness of privatization that were based on worse care only told part of the story. These explicit arguments concealed tacit recognitions of the NHS as a service whose good could only be evaluated on the basis of how it served the whole society, both as a provider of healthcare and as an employer. The NHS was an icon but also a material structure through which mutual responsibility was enacted. Therefore any reform which led to a diminishment in its provision of services or wages to one person or group should be contested as a moral failure, as an injury to all. The ethical unit of interest to them, enshrined in the NHS's aspiration to universality, was the whole population. This solidaristic view of the NHS was the implicit basis of NHS activism against privatization, not immediately noticeable in their explicit reasoning, but illuminated on deeper investigation. They converted these tacit moral frameworks to explicit outcomes-based arguments to fit a world in which Stephen Dorrell and his colleagues could only be swayed by 'what matters is what works'. Their collectivist ethics, in which everyone mattered, underlay the way in which they answered the practical question of what worked, allowing them to consider the proponents of privatization as immoral.

The vulnerability of the welfare state

Having now established the wrongness of privatization, and how activists explained that wrongness, I move on to the question of why their sensitivity to the possibility of privatization so often hardened into concrete predictions. I start by identifying the pattern that links the anti-privatization struggles described above. Describing the pattern will help to understand the moral argumentation of NHS activists. Activists are always on the lookout for routes through which private capital can make inroads into owning and running parts of the NHS. When they find such a route, they make predictions that the route will be followed, that is, they do not just point out that services *could* be privatized, but foresee that they *will* be privatized. Importantly, they are able to provide evidence for current predictions by looking to previous predictions that have come true. I paraphrase the basic argument here, amalgamating a few different quotations from Catherine, Olga and Nancy, taking the industrial dispute over Olga's dismissal as an example:

> At the time of the nurses' strike, we stated that more services would be outsourced in the future. Now look at addictions services, look at early intervention services,[31] look at the increasing use of private inpatient beds, look at services x, y and z that have – as we predicted – been privatized.

The thrust of the argument is that when there is a route for private capital to take control of a service, eventually that route is taken.

Spire's projection of expansion following NHS cuts (see Chapter 2) and Dorrell and Dunne's comments that there should be no barriers to further privatization underline the point that undergirds NHS activists' sense of fear around any new policy announcement: state welfare services *are* vulnerable.[32] Welfare is vulnerable to cuts because it is expensive and states that can provide the cheapest labour vie for advantage over other states when competing for capital investment. Welfare services are also vulnerable to privatization since capital continues to look for ways to reproduce itself, and state welfare represents a potential steady source of income in capitalist states. Whatever politicians and managers say, or even what they believe, capital's will to expand into spaces it has not yet colonized remains rapacious. Growth is inherent to the profit motive. The state has struggled to resist the interests of private industry generally, and private healthcare specifically.[33]

It was recognition of the vulnerability of the welfare state that led NHS activists' conjecture to harden into definite predictions. 'Could' turned to 'will' because state actors were powerless in the face of capital. When the money ran out, local managers had to get money from somewhere. From the 1980s onwards, money only came with strings attached in the form of private investment, for example, through Private Finance Initiatives. As Catherine told me in an interview,

> A lot of the managers didn't necessarily want to privatize things, but it's the only way they can run things. It's the only way they're going to get money from the government … So in a sense you can't blame them for doing it, they're making … quite logical decisions because that's the way they're being funded.

Catherine's quotation underlines the impossible position of the local manager. Even when they disagree with private involvement in healthcare, their hands are forced. They have to open themselves to private investment because as managers they have a responsibility to keep the service running. If the resources are not coming from central government, they have no other option.[34]

Take Wigan's senior manager who told me that activists talking about privatization were unhelpful, unrealistic conspiracy theorists. A few months later, he was a key player in the trust's attempted outsourcing of its staff to a subsidiary company. Either he was being disingenuous or naïve. But Blair's dictum can help us to understand his actions. 'What matters is what works.' His responsibility was not to the whole NHS, nor the whole population. Unlike activists' commitment to a broader sense of the good of the NHS as they imagined it, 'what works' for him incorporated a duty to balance the trust's books. He just needed to make sure that the organization continued to run, within the financial constraints that were set by the government, over which he had no control. If privatization of some aspects of the trust was what worked to keep it afloat, by way of reducing staff overheads, then it fitted with what Catherine described as 'the only way they can run things'.

Activists understood that the hands of state actors were tied. Since activists' fears and predictions of privatization hinged on a perception of the powerlessness of the state in the face of capital, we can interpret their moral arguments as a critique of capitalist social relations. The beliefs and discourse of the managers and politicians issuing policy documents did not reassure activists even if they stated that privatization was not the goal of any particular reform, as they did with LCOs in Manchester and ACOs in Dunning. Activists continued to search for ways that the reforms *could* lead to privatization. Any routes that were found crystallized into hard predictions – 'could' became 'would' – because they understood the state to no longer have the capacity to resist the inexorable expansion of private industry.

If state actors were weak in the face of capital, if privatization was almost inevitable, and if privatization was wrong, then the future was to be feared. But NHS activists had learnt privatization could be at least slowed, and in some cases stopped, by struggles motivated by fears of privatization. They gave me many examples of how they had slowed privatization over the years. The ones I have mentioned in this chapter have been their opposition to foundation trusts and the industrial action following Olga's dismissal. In both cases, activists felt that if they had not protested, there would have been more cuts and more privatization. In the case of the Wigan industrial dispute, the strike and picket had contributed to completely stopping that particular outsourcing. At least temporarily.

The effectiveness of NHS activism as a means of resisting privatization adds further texture to their subversion of the neoliberal logic of 'what matters is what works'. The social and historical context invoked by Dorrell when he used this quotation was that of an NHS in which New Public Management (NPM) had been consolidated over the previous decades.[35] Although NPM is often summarized as, 'what matters is what works', the aphorism does not capture NPM's failure to question the structural restraints imposed upon managers through its efficiency logic, the exact restraints that Catherine referred to when she said, 'A lot of the managers didn't necessarily want to privatize things, but it's the only way they can run things. It's the only way they're going to get money from the government'.

According to activists, public ownership 'worked' better than privatization, subverting the logic of NPM while fitting its rubric of what matters is what works. But more than that, NHS activism 'worked' – at least partially – to resist privatization. It was this double subversion of what matters is what works that I argue lubricated the transition from looking for ways that parts of the NHS could be privatized to predicting that there would be privatization. In the context of a temporality of fear, and an empirically grounded conviction that the state was powerless in the face of global capital, campaigning to resist privatization was galvanized by predictions that privatization would indeed take place. As a Socialist Party pamphlet that Leon gave me said, 'If we fight, we can win'. But we need to have something to fight first.

Operose and actually existing privatization

Developments since my fieldwork suggest that the activist critique of the vulnerability of the welfare state was well justified, and the temporality of fear was warranted. As elaborated in Chapter 2, privatization has continued, both as buy-out and sell-off. The £1.3bn contract for all community-based care in one Integrated Care Board in South West England, given to private company HCRG Care Group, itself owned by private equity firm

Twenty20Capital (Talora, 2024) has vindicated some of the fears that activists had around ACOs. As of April 2025, former NHS employees in the region are now directly employed by HCRG.

But what did activists miss?

I now elaborate the story of Operose's privatization of GP services in 2021 to illustrate where activists' critique was underdeveloped. To understand how it might be possible for their critique to have had this blind spot, given the overarching temporality of fear, I return to their understanding of the NHS as a moral example.

In 2020, the organization that Lemmy was concerned about, Centene, consolidated its subsidiaries into one company called Operose Health. By 2021, it already ran 20 GP practices (Davidson, 2021). It then acquired a further 37 surgeries in London, meaning the corporation was providing primary care for over 500,000 people.[36] As Chris Thomas (2022) observes, NHS activists were horrified. They objected, but by then it was too late. Thomas analyses how it was possible for such a large-scale privatization to take place without activists having been alert to the possibility *beforehand* and therefore able to mount a successful opposition. He describes the contractor model of general practice and how it came to be: a concession from Bevan in order to convince the BMA to accept the creation of the NHS in 1948.[37]

He argues that the contractor model made sense in 1948. But by the time Thomas wrote his book, general practice was widely accepted as being in crisis, with people around the country struggling to be able to see a GP, and GPs themselves struggling with workload. Thomas is understandably frustrated with NHS activists' tendency to be on the defensive rather than looking to:

> universalis[e] the best … rear-guard action forces us to wait until it happens, and only then react … We could have prevented privatisation by nationalising GPs … And yet … the idea of changing the model of general practice is fiercely opposed by the key institutions of the health labour movement: royal colleges and trade unions. Both are staunch defenders of the status quo in general practice, as broken as it is. Both put out media statements dismissing the nationalisation policy – six months later, Centene was the biggest GP operator in the country. (2022: 161–162)

Thomas did not do empirical research with activists themselves. My research may be better placed to shed light on the question of how activists' temporality of fear missed this pathway to privatization that, in hindsight, seems obvious. As described above, the activists I spent time with were largely – although not entirely – relaxed regarding the prevailing structure of general practice. Their fears were focused on the new changes being brought in rather than the structures that had existed since 1948.

In Chapter 1, I demonstrated how activists understood the NHS as a moral example of socialism, to be protected *as such*. However, when asked directly what was wrong with privatization, their explicit arguments appeared consequentialist and utilitarian. Although it might be possible to build a socialist politics from a utilitarian ethics, I also demonstrated how other scraps of moral argumentation emerged from broader examination of their discourse and actions, demonstrating how their manifestation of a socialist politics did not, in fact, rely only on utilitarian reasoning. Instead, an understanding of solidarity within a broad community of interest was implicit in their choices to protest with NHS workers. As described in Chapter 1, the moral example combined a perception of the material institution of the NHS as a manifestation of mutual obligation within society – actually existing socialism – with an understanding that the existing institution was not, in fact, realizing this aspiration.

However, the temporality of fear was focused on the dangers posed by reforms. That is, activists were looking out for how managers and politicians were attempting to bring about changes that would create pathways to privatization. The most worrying threats were those that lurked around the corner, in the future, rather than those enduring from the NHS's imagined socialist origins. Activists' attention was not on which pathways were embedded in the founding of the NHS. I argue that this oversight was related to the use of the NHS as an example and a template to assess what might be wrong with contemporary plans to change it. What was good about the NHS was precisely the fact that it provided healthcare that was universal, free and comprehensive. Its material structure was what made it good. Changes to its material structure were exactly what was to be opposed.

Although Chris Thomas, a trained economist working for a think tank, did diagnose a material and structural weakness not just in proposed reforms, but also within the *existing* structure of the NHS, activists were somewhat blinded by the indexing of the moral example of socialism with the structure forged by Bevan. As described by Webb Keane (2010), moral reasoning is not an abstract, ideal or transcendent process that determines our actions in the real, material world. Instead moral values are embodied in everyday practices, material objects and public performances (see also Keane, 2007). In this case, the particular institutional form that NHS values were embedded in was its 1948 structure. The NHS *was* good, in every sense of the word, and activists felt it ought to be defended, with that defence forming part of their identity as socialists. This reasoning remained implicit. If I ever asked if the NHS of 1948 was perfect, they would say no, it was simply a template to work on. And yet, their values – universal, free, comprehensive – were hitched to their imagination of that materiality. Thus, in their moral subjectivities, there was 'a sharpening of ethical awareness' (Keane, 2010: 72) around reforms, manifesting in the temporality of fear. But this hitching of

NHS values to a pre-existing structure also obscured a deeper materialist analysis of where, how and why the NHS failed to realize its aspirations, since attention was focused on the – very real – dangers posed by people and organizations seeking to reform those structures.

Conclusion

This chapter has made two key arguments. First, I have demonstrated how activists' explicit arguments regarding the wrongness of privatization presupposed a different ethical unit of interest from Stephen Dorrell and other advocates of privatization: everyone in the UK rather than any one particular individual. Unpicking the focus on worse outcomes through the rubric of 'what matters is what works' revealed how their arguments were undergirded by a perception of the implicit moral system of the NHS as an example of how a state could intervene in society to provide a structure through which all of its members' interests would be protected.

Second, sustained attention on the rubric of 'what matters is what works' has allowed me to explain why activists' searching for potential paths to privatization so often crystallized into hard predictions. Such predictions grounded a critique of the vulnerability of the welfare state, thus facilitating political struggles to save it. Activists had memories of these struggles working to slow privatization, something that state actors were themselves unable to do.

I have added further texture to the role of the NHS in the temporalities of NHS activists. I started with Ronny's puzzle of why some activists see privatization everywhere. In following the process from the wrongness of privatization through to empirical evidence that grounds activists' ever-present fear of privatization, I illustrated that in their temporality, the future is to be feared. Privatization is always on the horizon, because contemporary state actors have few other means of making their organizations work. States are weak compared to global capital. But NHS activists *have* resisted privatization, and they remember their struggles as at least partially successful. These 'collective memories of struggle' (Schmidt, 2015: 30) add another layer of meaning to the symbolism of the NHS.

However, I also highlighted one place that activists did not look for pathways to privatization: in the origin story of the NHS. Recognition of our shared interests was given institutional form in the moral example of the NHS. Therefore, insults to that material form represented ethical threats. Activists understood reforms as dangerous, and the ongoing privatization of large sections of the NHS demonstrates how they activists fears were justified. However, the advance of privatization in areas where many activists did *not* anticipate it demonstrates how their critique of the state's vulnerability was underdeveloped.

I have argued that this blind spot was inherently linked to their conceptualization of the NHS as a moral example. Their moral framework – built on their interpretation of the material structure of the NHS – affected where they devoted their attention, their implicit reasoning did not remain internal but had effects on their actions, and thus had rebound consequences for the materiality of the institution they sought to defend. The next chapter builds on the consequences that flowed from their moral reasoning, focusing more on group formation.

4

Whose Side are NHS Managers on?

Content warning – suicide

In April 2018, I attended a talk given by Ronny at the Dunning Labour Club.[1] His lecture was entitled, 'How did the NHS get to be like this?' I sat next to Esther, who was sitting next to one of the Dunning councillors whom I had interviewed, Brian. They knew each other because Esther was also a member of the Labour Party. Esther was warm and congenial, as usual, but Brian seemed a little cold. There were several other members of Dunning KONP present. They all knew who Brian was, but they sat on the other side of the room from him.

Everyone was quiet for the talk. At times, I noticed Dunning KONP members grimacing at parts with which they disagreed. Brian sat completely still, arms crossed, eyes straight ahead.

Afterwards, Ronny opened the floor to questions. A few of the Dunning KONP members made comments that hinted at their reservations regarding current NHS reforms in Dunning and nationally. Then one of them, Alan, stood up and said, 'It seems like the starting point of what is happening now is not how do we redesign things to improve services to help people, but how do we redesign services to save money'. To my left, I was aware of other Dunning KONP members either nodding or bristling with shared anger, agreeing with Alan. To my right, Brian finally showed some emotion. He was also angry, but unlike the activists, he disagreed with Alan. Under his breath, I heard him mutter, 'That's not true.' I did not hear him say anything else during the meeting.

A few months earlier, in October 2017, I had interviewed Brian with another Dunning councillor, Theo. They both expressed their frustration with the members of Dunning KONP with whom they were clashing. Based on what they had said to me in the interview, I suggested to them that perhaps their understandings of the values of the NHS were not so different from Dunning KONP members'. Both Brian and Theo agreed. Brian said, 'I don't think we're far apart. It's just: how do we get there?'

In this chapter, I pose the disagreements between activists and state actors as a puzzle. The puzzle that quickly came to light in my fieldwork was that the actors involved on both sides of this clash described the values of the NHS in the same terms, centring around the maxim: 'universal, free and comprehensive'. How could it be that they agreed on the values of the NHS, and yet were engaged in a battle regarding how it should be structured?

I attempt to solve this puzzle through reference to what I will call ideological closure: the narrowing of available options for the solution of a problem. This closure consisted in the enclosure of managers' ethical reasoning within financial constraints, and the use of these constraints to foreclose political debate. Activists sought to mobilize various forms of accountability to prise open the enclosure and to counter the foreclosure. At times activists were successful; managers and politicians were swayed by or simply agreed with activists. However, managers mostly did so quietly, not allowing themselves to be deterred from the reforms they were enacting.

The dynamic at play for these managers was what I call corporate accountability, an upwards accountability to one's employer. I will demonstrate how this form of accountability amounted to a coercion that placed limits on the moral reasoning and political action of these managers. Rather than the well-trodden story of a trend of audit and numerical accounting trumping and subsuming other forms of accountability (Strathern, 1997; 2000b; Shore and Wright, 2015),[2] I argue that managers had to be *forced* to place limits on their moral responsibilities. That is, I describe a process of coercion rather than Foucauldian disciplining. Rather than spontaneously justifying the cuts which they were administering as necessary for the organization to function within its allocated budgets, they had to be corralled into seeing their pecuniary responsibility as over-riding other obligations, such as to provide high-quality health services for all. Audit was not the only technology through which the neoliberal reconfiguration of state welfare services was driven. Corporate accountability was the means by which financial accountability's primacy was maintained.

The structure of the chapter is as follows: I begin by reviewing the literature on audit and accountabilities. I follow the oft-recounted story of the redefinition of responsibility in the neoliberal state (Rose, 1992), and New Public Management's role in this redefinition (Hood and Dixon, 2015). Power's (1999; 2000) era-defining work on 'audit society' and Strathern's (Strathern, 2000a) collection on 'audit cultures' followed Rose (1992) and were the foundations for anthropological studies of accountability. Shore and Wright (2015) and Trnka and Trundle (2017) have been among those who have documented a story of the gradual eclipsing of political accountability by the importance of financial accountability.

I then elucidate how my ethnographic material adds further complexity to contemporary understandings of accountability. Unlike the dual credentials of accountability noted by Strathern (2000b), in moral reasoning and financial accounting, goodness and efficiency, I found multiple dimensions of accountability being mobilized by my interlocutors, overlapping and interacting with one another. In the heady mix of accountabilities that I will describe, I will demonstrate how certain power dynamics stood out and gave order to the mess. Namely, accountability to a perceived centre of governance in London over-rode all other accountabilities. Or to put it another way, the space within which managers and politicians were able to use their own ethical sensibilities – perhaps following a sense of duty to represent constituents, or obligation to provide state services to citizens – to counter the logic of audit was severely limited by their fear that they would get sacked. Some of my interlocutors *did* get sacked, precisely for speaking out against cuts or reforms that they argued were caused by cuts.

The fact that some managers spoke out while others did not, and some managers lost their jobs while others did not, points to the uneven forces at play. Separating the different forms of accountability will help to make sense not just of the ideological closure of managers and politicians, but also their discourse around it. Put simply, they trumpeted the positive aspects of change and muted the risks *because they had to*. If they did not, they feared they would be held accountable by their employer; they would lose their jobs.

Managers, politicians and ideological closure

When I interviewed Dunning councillors, Brian and Theo, they expressed the view that, far from being a route to the destruction of the NHS, the plans to rationalize hospital services and improve community services in Dunning were, in fact, the only way to save the NHS. They expressed their frustration with the members of Dunning KONP with whom, in their words, they were 'clashing', since the activists were getting in the way of the politicians' rescue mission. Brian and Theo explained to me that they held to the NHS's values, and that their goal was to improve the health of Dunning's citizens, reducing inequality in the process. To maintain the NHS – and NHS values – they had to respond to the real circumstances with which they were faced: demand for healthcare was increasing, just as the resources available were reducing. Drastically. If they did not act, then the gap between demand and available resources would only increase: 'We estimate that by 2020, if we don't do anything with new models of care and reforms, the gap between what it would cost to provide health and social care … and the resources available would be about £130m.'

The councillors were all too aware that their budget was insufficient, and that it had been handed down to them by a central government that they felt was seeking to devolve not power, but blame. They told me that if inadequate resources led to worse health services, it would be the local politicians that would be held responsible by voters. However, they still felt that the reforms they were pushing through were the best way to get as close to a realization of NHS values as possible, within the constraints set by finite resources.

Following their lead, I asked all of the councillors I met if they considered affordability or efficiency as themselves ethical principles. Generally, they did not, when I phrased a direct question in that way. A senior Labour councillor in another part of Manchester, Niamh, gave me a typical response when she described the requirement to spend within one's means as 'the reality'. Niamh put it to me that efficiency was not in itself an ethical principle that she held to, but that she did seek to do the best for the NHS with what was 'within our gift'. In reference to the £6bn allocated to all of Greater Manchester for the NHS, the Leader of another council in Greater Manchester, Paul, said to me, 'No, it's not enough in a sense, but it's what we've got. That's the thing … so we need to find ways of making sure that money is well used, better used, more effectively addressing the needs of populations rather than simply providing ill-health care.'

I am not seeking to say that efficiency had not crept into their ethics. Indeed, other statements regarding a responsibility to be careful with 'taxpayers' money' did suggest that they understood economic prudence to be one of the duties of 'decision makers with budgetary responsibility working in the public sector'. Regardless, ethics can be *debated*. The point I am arguing here is that managers and politicians did not regard the finitude of their resources as something they could debate. It was simply a *reality* that formed the constraints within which they had to act. Any values they had could only be realized as far as was possible within those constraints. As Prime Minister Theresa May said in 2017, 'there is no magic money tree'.[3] Get used to it. Put otherwise, once councillors and managers have accepted that the money they are given is what they have got, parsimony becomes unavoidable. There is no debate.

In the eyes of managers and politicians, they had formed a plan to do the best they could with 'what we've got'. Since Dunning KONP were seeking to stop the council from taking these actions, councillors began to see them as adversaries. It was NHS activists that were stopping councillors from realizing the values of the NHS. In opposing NHS reforms, councillors felt that the activists were 'trouble-makers', advocating a 'do-nothing scenario' that would ultimately lead to the collapse of the NHS. I saw councillors become visibly angry when discussing Dunning KONP. Theo banged his hand on the table in the middle of the interview with me. Another shouted at Dunning KONP aggressively during a public engagement event that I had organized. Dunning KONP members told me about other incidents of verbal abuse they had received from Dunning's councillors. These councillors justified their actions to evade or shut down negotiation with NHS activists on the basis that it was the activists that were getting in the way of managers and politicians realizing the values of the NHS *as far as was possible*.

What was possible was limited by 'what we've got'. The managers and politicians I spoke to were not comfortable with the financial constraints that they had to deal with; they wished that they had more money. But they did accept the constraints as realities within which they had to work, and to make the NHS work. My contention is not that state actors did not have ethical aspirations. As Bear and Mathur (2015) have highlighted, bureaucrats' utopian aspirations and the ways in which they do or do not act to realize them can be fruitful terrain to analyse the pressures at play for social groups, including the bureaucrats themselves. I found that managers and politicians often used the same ethical discourse as activists to describe the values of the NHS and underpin their political action: 'free, universal, comprehensive'. However, managers and politicians sought to realize these values within the financial constraints that were the precise point of contention for campaigners.

Activists took financial constraints and spoke about their morality, in order to expose them to debate. They made the technocratic moral in order to make it political. They did this by arguing that proposed reforms would result in foregoing the state's obligations to its citizens. Managers claimed to have the same values as activists, but sought to narrow the space within which moral judgements could be made, in order to confine the space of political debate. Bureaucrats had already decided what was possible within *enclosed* limits. Further challenges to their plans were to be shut down. Debate was *foreclosed*.

I call this placement of boundaries around what was achievable ideological closure. Giving it a name begs the question: what drove the ideological closure of these managers? The word, closure, suggests resolution, as in the closure sought after the end of an intimate relationship. But this chapter will describe closure as a process. I will describe how processes of enclosure and foreclosure facilitated ideological closure, tending towards but never quite achieving resolution, leaving cracks open for the ethical imagination of the people charged with administering audit practices. The argument of this chapter is that, sometimes, they had to be coerced to constrain their moral arguments against service retrenchment, to deem their responsibility to spend within their allocated budgets as more important than other responsibilities.

Anthropological literature on accountability

Anthropological studies of accountability have focused on audit cultures, defined by Shore and Wright as 'the widespread proliferation of … calculative rationalities of modern financial accounting and their effects on individuals and organizations' (2015: 421). Shore and Wright follow a Foucauldian framework in which they expose a regime of truth in which quantitative indicators and measurements have become increasingly pervasive in the organizations they investigated: universities. These measurements became important both as instruments for universities to use within their own internal governance, but also in their external representations of quality and efficiency, aspects of their accountability to the public, to employees and to students. The transparent exposition of such measures was supposed to demonstrate best practice to these stakeholders, who would thus have the means by which to hold the university to account.

Shore and Wright were interested not just in how audit culture reshaped organizational accountability, but also in audit as a totalizing technology of contemporary life that had become widely institutionalized through the practices of 'New Public Management' (NPM), from the 1980s onwards. NPM's use of audit encouraged staff and students not just to understand the accountability of the university in terms of measurable outcomes, but also to apply the same understanding to themselves as individuals. Staff were encouraged to understand their responsibilities as employees through a prism of accountability that could be conceived through calculable inputs and outputs, for which they were responsible as academic workers.

As political and managerial processes were reshaping individual subjectivities in this way, ranking technologies were reshaping the organization and work of universities according to whatever was being ranked. Thus audit became inescapable as the pursuit of good practice – measured by pre-set quantitative outcomes, to be transparently assessed, recorded and presented – became self-justifying, even as it over-rode and stripped away professional autonomy. Shore and Wright (2015: 422) drew a comparison with Weber's iron cage of bureaucracy, instead referring to audit as the glass cage of coercive transparency.[4] However, this was not literal coercion, but a quasi-coercion through disciplinary processes; the responsible subject was both being formed and (re)forming herself, auditing herself in cognizance of being audited by her superiors.[5]

For Shore and Wright, audit is a top-down technology of accountability, 'as those in positions of power seek to make legible the performance of those below them' (2015: 429). The auditees, in this case professional academics, object to the obvious imbalance of transparency and accountability by invoking their professional ethics. But as Strathern (2000b) noted, and as Shore and Wright reiterate, managerial indicators were often very difficult to oppose precisely because they co-opt and redefine professional values such as responsibility, quality, self-management and transparency.

Teghtsoonian raised the puzzle of the audit juggernaut: if it is neither totalizing, nor particularly effective at even achieving its explicit goals (such as improved quality or efficiency of delivered services), then why do governments and managers continue to have faith in it? (See Hood and

Dixon, 2015, for evidence in relation to NPM in the UK.) This chapter provides one response to this puzzle. Managers stick to audit practices because they are forced to by their own managers.

Social policy and health services literature

Day and Klein's (1987) history of accountabilities in public services is now almost 40 years old, but its conceptualization of the state remains a useful point of departure:

> The modern Welfare State is also the service-delivery State. Its development has compounded the problems of making those who deliver services answerable both to those who finance them and those who use them ... as the systems of service delivery have become more complex, so it has become more difficult to assign responsibility ... Yet if there is a great deal of interest in accountability, there is a great deal of confusion about what this chameleon word means. (1987: 1)

In this conceptualization of the state, certain actors are responsible for delivering a suite of services within a budget set by their superiors. These state actors may fail in their responsibilities (e.g. to a promise, or to uphold their own duties or professional ethics, or simply to balance the books). But being held accountable for such a failure would be a separate step that implies a *relationship* (to a person or electorate, to a regulatory body, or to an auditor/line manager). Day and Klein attributed these changing relationships, and an increasing interest in these forms of accountability, to the transformation of the welfare state to the service delivery state, in which managers and politicians had to find ways to stretch increasingly limited resources to provide the services expected by citizens.

Day and Klein discuss the techniques of audit – performance indicators, targets, outcome assessments – that later crystallized under NPM, defined by Hood and Dixon as a 'a set of loosely related ideas about government and public service reform ... ostensibly intended to create "a government that works better and costs less"' (2015: 265). Hood and Dixon (Hood, 2010; Hood and Dixon, 2015) were among many (Hewison, 2002; e.g. Bezes et al, 2012) who researched NPM and found negative consequences in terms of the outputs of the organizations involved: lower productivity, increased costs, more complaints. But scholarly critique of NPM did not slow it down; NPM continued to expand within the NHS throughout the 1990s and 2000s, closely tied to the politics of neoliberalism. Although social policy and health service researchers such as Day, Klein and Hood often focused on organizational outcomes rather than individual subjectivities, the structural processes they were observing were the same ones that Shore and

Wright (2015) investigated in universities. Audit and financial accountability became the means by which neoliberal reforms were effected in many state and state-funded structures, including healthcare, social services, schools and higher education.

At the same time as the flourishing of NPM, the complexity of the organization of service provision also continued to increase.[6] Central government remains nominally in control of the overall function of the NHS, supposedly to be held to account at general elections. When a central body is supposed to be in charge of a number of different organizational actors, questions are raised as to how and when to exert or threaten hierarchical control. Health services researchers have investigated these questions internationally and found that the difficulty in making such judgements has led to 'pendulum swings' (Axelsson, 2000: 47) between central control and decentralization. Hammond et al (2018: 1151), investigating the purported swing back towards decentralization in the NHS at the time of my fieldwork, note that '[s]uch attempts to redistribute power from central government to agencies and localities provide fertile conditions for "blame games" (Hood, 2010), "buck-passing", and accountability ambiguity when objectives are not met'.

The focus of Hammond et al's study is NHS England, an arms-length body set up by the Health and Social Care Act 2012, ostensibly to allow the NHS to be run by experts with a long-term mandate, rather than being subject to 'political interference' or 'micro-management' by meddling MPs with short-term electoral goals.[7] However, health ministers continued to influence NHS England (Timmins, 2018), albeit in the absence of transparency. Hammond et al (2018) found multiple formal and contractual technologies of accountability *upwards* to NHS England, such as assurance demands, the NHS Outcomes Framework and key performance indicators. As a result of these measures, bureaucrats working in local organizations such as CCGs described their experience in terms of constraint rather than the autonomy that might be expected with decentralization. On the other hand, accountability *downwards* to patients and public was more limited and unclear.

Hammond et al found that rather than protecting the NHS from government, NHS England served to 'insulate government ministers from unpopular policies, thus shifting, or obscuring, the locus of accountability' (2018: 1152). Government set the 'rules of the game' (Hammond et al, 2018: 1148), but it was NHS England that enforced the rules. In so doing, NHS England highlighted the difference between responsibility and accountability, as well as the political importance of such a difference. That is, while government ultimately was responsible for many of the decisions that were driving changes to the NHS, NHS England obscured how people *related* to it, and thus how they could hold it accountable. Providers of care had a direct relationship to NHS England rather than to government, and accountability mechanisms worked through that relationship. Since the accountability relationship with government was unclear, Hammond et al argued that a process of 'depoliticisation' (2018: 1163) was taking place. Government was creating policies and driving transformations, and people's contestation of such reforms was defanged by government's insulation by NHS England.

These papers have established the wider context. My ethnographic account will go into more detail on how people were experiencing the above processes and how they mobilized various meanings of accountability in their contestation of particular transformations. Activists were deeply frustrated by managers and politicians failing to acknowledge responsibility for their decisions and actions. Members of Dunning KONP and Greater Manchester KONP could see that the NHS was struggling, that the services being offered were diminishing and deteriorating, they predicted that further cuts and privatization would make things even worse, and they wanted to hold someone accountable for these undesired happenings. Meanwhile, they heard managers and politicians at all levels speak only about the achievements of the NHS, and the positive results of current and future reforms, not the negative consequences that exercised activists.

Accountability as answerability

In the eyes of campaigners, the people most responsible for NHS reforms were the Tory national government and the senior managers in London that had been appointed by that government. Although they spoke of holding those politicians accountable, they were aware that the primary mechanism for democratic accountability of Westminster politicians came at general elections. That would mean waiting several years, during which time the same politicians continued to exert an influence over the NHS that these activists considered to be malign. Frequently, I heard them say, 'We cannot wait for an election'.

Of course, democratic accountability does not only manifest at elections. Activists and other members of the public expected MPs to answer for their actions and inactions, to show that they had understood the consequences thereof. To illustrate this type of accountability – as answerability – I describe a public meeting organized by Bolton KONP in November 2017, at which a panel of mental health professionals, activists and service users spoke to residents of the area. One person on the panel was a mother, Jess, who spoke of the tragic death of her son, Jordan. He had sought help at the local emergency department when he felt suicidal. After waiting for three hours, he had been assessed by a mental health practitioner and then discharged with no follow-up arranged. A few weeks later, his suicidal thoughts returned. He went to a park and ended his life.

The organizer of the meeting, Olga, was herself a mental health nurse, as well as a union and KONP activist. After the mother had finished speaking, Olga said to the audience:

> You may be thinking: how could this happen? Actually, this kind of story is far from exceptional. It happens far too often. We are the fifth richest country in the world. We are not a poor country. But we choose to starve our NHS, especially mental health, so much that we have such a poor service that people's experience is such that they end up in this kind of situation.

Rather than focus on the role of the clinician who saw Jordan, or the clinician's managers, Olga allocated responsibility upwards, to the government that had made fiscal decisions that shaped the environment in which that clinician worked. She did implicitly acquiesce to a sense that the trust was at fault, but also pointed towards the many other people failed by trusts across the country. How could this happen? Because trusts did not have enough money to employ enough staff. And responsibility for that lack of funds lay with the national government. People like Jordan were suffering the consequences for decisions taken by politicians in Westminster.

Olga's allocation of responsibility upwards created a moral antagonist: the Tory government. In creating a moral antagonist, she positioned herself as in alliance with Jess, and with users or potential users of the NHS more broadly. Bolton had a Tory MP who had voted for many of the cuts that people were angry about. Therefore, Olga suggested that on Saturday, we march to his office for his weekly constituency surgery. The plan was to explain the story to him, since

> He should know what he's signing his name to when he says the health service can't have any more money. When people walk away from services because they can't face the wait, because of what he has done, he should face that. He should know what he's doing. It's heartbreaking when you hear that, isn't it? He should hear that.

It was clear to Olga that the MP was at least partially responsible for this death, as well as many others. But until he acknowledged his responsibility, until he was made to *answer* for his failure to uphold that responsibility, he had not been *held to account*. Holding him to account in this way, following a march in concert with others, was a strategy that could consolidate the alliance of people who understood their relation to the state as one that was being undermined by a failed obligation, manifesting in inadequate funds and thus inadequate care, 'because of what he [the Tory MP] has done'. Thus they were holding him to account for a failed responsibility of the state that they were reproducing and reinforcing as they alluded to it.

Similarly, in January 2018, Olga brought an academic paper (Hiam et al, 2017) to a Greater Manchester KONP meeting that attributed responsibility for 30,000 excess deaths in 2015 to cuts in health and social care. She was frustrated that the government had not been held accountable for these deaths. The purpose of the march – as well as actions that she proposed following the publication of the academic paper – was to communicate a sense of that responsibility both to the government itself, and to a wider public, as well as to demand an explanation. Any answer that prioritized balancing budgets over human lives would be inadequate; such an answer would be morally wrong. But the important point for accountability was to *get* an explicit answer.

Accountability as transparency

Getting an answer implies asking a question. But activists often told me that part of what was so troubling about recent reforms of the NHS wasn't just the cuts and privatization, but that it was so difficult to work out *what* had been cut or privatized. Thus the question itself was difficult to formulate. The Health and Social Care Act 2012 had not just made the division of NHS structures more complex. The new commissioning arrangements meant that it was often very difficult for someone to know which of their local NHS services were no longer being provided, being provided with a reduced remit, with fewer staff, or by a private company. Moreover, any contract that an organization held to provide a service to the NHS would not be visible to the public. It would be protected by commercial confidentiality. But the complexity of the contracts and the dynamic ecology of service provision did not just make healthcare structures unintelligible for activists, patients and citizens. Politicians also found it difficult to keep up with how the NHS worked, and how it was changing. Almost every MP and councillor I spoke to admitted to not fully understanding the NHS.[8]

The relative ignorance of councillors was a recurring theme among the activists that I spent time with. Activists oscillated between a desire to ally with, educate and help these politicians to understand current and future structures, and exasperation at councillors resisting their explanations and offers of help. Meanwhile, councillors ploughed on with the reforms that campaigners felt would facilitate privatization. Dunning KONP and Greater Manchester KONP members knew that the chief architects of reforms were in London, people like then Secretary of State for Health and Social Care, Jeremy Hunt, and then Chief Executive of NHS England, Simon Stevens. But they had no avenues through which to engage with Westminster managers and politicians. They could only engage with – to hold accountable – the people with whom they had more of a relationship, local managers and politicians. Hence their vexation when these people did not acknowledge the risks that activists explained to them, instead focusing on the need for reforms, which they trumpeted as positive changes.

When I spoke to managers and politicians privately, they *did* acknowledge that responding to budgetary constraints was a key driver for the reforms they were advocating, because limited finances were simply 'the reality'. They also acknowledged the risks that activists voiced. But they did so quietly, without allowing the acknowledgement of such risks to deter their path.

Nor did managers and politicians often speak about cutting hospitals as a goal of reforms. This lack of explicitness was part of what activists referred to when they said the plans were far from transparent. On the rare occasions when politicians *were* explicit regarding such plans, activists were shocked. One member of Dunning KONP, Debbie, told me several times of when she heard a senior Manchester councillor speaking at an NHS Innovation conference. She shuddered in disbelief when he said that he looked forward to a time when Manchester would be able to 'reduce its hospital provision', that is, to shut hospitals. I asked that councillor about this when I interviewed him. He explained the same arguments that I had heard from managers and politicians around the city: that hospitals were bad places for people to recover from illness, due to the risks of muscle-wasting, of hospital-acquired infections, of iatrogenic injury. It would be better for patients, as well as cheaper, to treat those people in their own homes.

I replied, 'I think everyone would probably welcome a service that was able to keep people out of hospital … I think the anxiety [of activists] is that the hospital beds might be cut before we've got to –'.

He cut me off to say, 'Yeah, I understand that. The purpose, as part of the … scheme in agreeing the Transformation Fund, was basically to establish double-running so that we could set up the new services at the same time as the old services continuing to run, to basically address that question quite directly.' He was referring to a time-limited pot of money that had been allocated to Greater Manchester by NHS England to allow it to set up new community services at the same time as still running the hospital services. The fund was for £450m, ending in 2021. The theory was that while there was still money in the pot, there would be no need to close hospitals. Thus there would be enough time for the community services to be fully established, and reduce demand for hospital beds before those beds were lost.

I wondered about the fears of activists and professionals (e.g. Royal College of Emergency Medicine, 2017), that the presence of these new community services would not actually reduce demand for hospital services. I asked, 'And if, when the Transformation Fund comes to an end, when it's run out of money, community services have been upgraded and that hasn't reduced demand on hospital beds, what happens then?'

He replied, 'Yeah, we're in the shit.'[9]

When pushed, managers and politicians had to acknowledge the risks to which they were exposing the NHS. So why were they taking these risks, and doing so without full explanation to the public? If their actions were driven by an ideological closure in which they accepted fiscal austerity as simply 'the reality', rather than a political decision that could be contested, that does not explain the part that really annoyed NHS activists: managers and politicians' unerring public positivity regarding current NHS reforms and their reluctance to speak out regarding the inadequate funds for either maintaining the service as it was, or for carrying out the kind of reforms they were advocating.

Corporate accountability

One of the first managers that I interviewed was Betty, in Dunning. We arranged the interview at such a time that I could go straight from the weekly Dunning KONP protest. I walked into the hospital, looked for the signs directing me to the department where she sat and then walked up. Security had to let me through a couple of locked doors and then I got to the top floor, which felt very separate from the clinical areas; tidy, quiet and carpeted. One receptionist welcomed me and asked if I wanted a drink, which was an experience I was not used to in a hospital. Surprised by the offer, I declined and sat on the sofa in the waiting area, inspecting the magazines, which were all copies of *Public Sector Focus*. I read the byline on the cover: 'Public Sector Focus is aimed at decision makers with budgetary responsibility working in the public sector.' While I flicked through the magazine, I heard a somewhat frantic phone call taking place down the corridor. The receptionist had informed me that Betty was running a bit behind schedule, and I wondered if it was Betty that I could hear on the phone.

She eventually emerged and apologized profusely. She shook my hand and offered me a coffee again. Aware of time and the evident stress in her voice, I declined and we went into her office. She explained that she was extremely busy at the moment because of the 'PR disaster' that was the Accident & Emergency situation, which was what she was trying to sort out on the phone while I waited outside. NHS England had decided, 'in the spirit of openness and transparency', she said sarcastically, to publish every trust's Accident & Emergency four-hour data[10] every week over winter. Dunning were near the bottom the previous week, and likely to be near the bottom again that week. So she had lots to deal with. When we started the interview, she expanded further on these issues.

> The big thing at the moment that we're dealing with is the huge pressures that we're facing because of winter, with the number of

> patients needing to come into hospital, with the beds all being full. So there's lots of implications about that, political, media, all sorts. We're also … dealing with the fact that we have huge financial problems. We're almost going bankrupt, we have massive deficits and – again – the political and the strategic consequences of that. We're dealing at the moment with big, big changes that are happening in Dunning where we're trying to do more out of hospital care because we cannot carry on the way we are. So we're getting this big impact on patients and staff.

Activists feared that financial constraints were impacting patient services. Here Betty confirmed that fear. Activists also feared that in their public discourse regarding the changes being implemented in response to such financial constraints, managers were not being completely honest regarding the possible consequences. Again, Betty confirmed to me that activists were correct in this belief. First, she explained the reasons why current reconfigurations might benefit patients, namely that integration of healthcare and social care could reduce separation between services, thus allowing them to run together with fewer disruptions. Then she explained the problems:

> I think there is a dishonesty about how it's being presented to the public because we're not also talking enough about the fact that this is because we haven't got enough money to continue as we are. So I think what we're trying to do is good, but I don't know how honest the conversation is because we're not talking about the fact that we haven't got enough money and that's part of the reason for wanting to do this … So, we're only talking about the bit we want to talk about, packaging it up in a really positive way and therefore, understandably, it's leading to cynicism from these protest groups because we're not explaining it clearly and openly and as honestly as we should, in my view.

Moreover, she felt that managers at board level in the hospital trust and the other NHS organizations in Dunning had 'ignored Dunning KONP, kept them at arm's length, patronized them, criticized them and tried to stifle and stem discussion with them'.

Trying to make sense of her candidness, my thoughts went to Bob Kerslake. In December 2017, just before I interviewed Betty, Sir Bob Kerslake had quit his role as chair of King's College Hospital board in London. Kerslake, a life peer in the House of Lords and former Head of the Civil Service, was a well-known figure in the UK. His departure made the national newspapers, not least because he wrote an article in *The Guardian* (2017), entitled: 'I'm quitting as a hospital boss: dire NHS funding problems give me no choice'. The subtitle read: 'Our deficit at King's College hospital, London, means we will be put into financial special measures, while what the NHS really needs is a fundamental rethink'.

I asked Betty about her thoughts on Kerslake's very public resignation. Betty told me:

> I was just cheering him on, and I think lots of people were in the [health service] … I think if we're all honest, we're all cheering him on! Cheering him on because we agreed with everything he said. But none of us are going to [speak out ourselves] because we all want to keep our jobs, and not get into trouble. And we're not able to resign like him.

Betty and her colleagues could not be open with the public and with Dunning KONP regarding the risks that the NHS was being exposed to, because that would expose her own job to risk. She had a mortgage and children to consider. I describe the dynamic at play for Betty as corporate accountability, an upwards accountability to one's employer.

I learnt more about how this threat of losing one's job loomed over managers' decisions regarding their own discourse from Julian, a doctor as well as a senior manager in Dunning. Shortly before I interviewed him, he had been called to give evidence to Dunning Council's Health and Social Care Scrutiny Committee. At the meeting, he had said that cuts to the public health budget were irrational and went against the council's stated strategy of keeping people well in the community and thus reducing demand for hospital beds. Reducing spending would have a deleterious effect on population health. Members of Dunning KONP had been present at the meeting and had reported his comments back to other members. The next time Dunning KONP members went to a council cabinet meeting, with the Leader of Dunning Council present, they used the opportunity to ask him a question in which they directly quoted Julian.

In my interview with Julian, he told me that his frank criticism of public health budget cuts had led to some friction that led him to believe that his job was now in jeopardy. I told him that Dunning KONP had directly quoted him in their communication with the Leader, and he described such communication as 'eminently appropriate … It probably does not help enamour me to the Leader, but nonetheless, it's something that they are absolutely entitled to do. I mean, there would be no point in claiming a freedom to speak if people didn't have a right to quote you.' Julian had a very acute sense of the conflicting accountabilities in his professional life. He was aware of his corporate accountability to his employer, as well as his professional accountability to his patients. As a public health consultant, his patients were effectively the whole population of Dunning. He summarized the situation:

> I am accountable for my management decisions to my line manager in the council, to the Chief Executive. That's not in question. And [as] a manager, you have to do what the organization requires you to do. That's quite clear. It's the role of advising the public that's the issue because there, I see myself as a doctor advising a population and … I'm accountable to that population.

However, unlike hospital doctors who have direct encounters with their patients, he did not meet his patients. Therefore, it was not clear how they might hold him accountable. The regulator for doctors, the General Medical Council (GMC), stipulated what his professional duties were, and could hold him accountable to those duties.[11] But he felt his responsibility to protect and promote the health of Dunning's population went beyond just what the GMC said. Thus his professional ethics were enforced not just through upwards accountability to the GMC, but also through his own conscience, his sense of obligation and duty:

> As far as giving professionally correct advice to the population, and as far as giving professionally correct advice to the agencies that serve the population, that is something that I think I have an obligation to do. And I don't accept that I'm accountable to anybody for it … I think duty is more important than accountability.

Although he had initially told me that he was accountable to the population, he was very aware that this downwards accountability was impossible for that population to enforce. Thus it could easily be overridden by his upwards accountability to his employer. Having noted this possibility, he was able to protect and prioritize his obligation to the people through moral reasoning that relied on an institution other than accountability: professional ethics.

However, this process of moral reasoning was still vulnerable. He told me, 'if you have a duty to give advice, then the ideal is that your organization accepts that and therefore it doesn't create any conflict between that duty and [corporate] accountability'. But in his career, he recalled eight times when duty and accountability came into conflict, placing his employment in peril. Unlike other managers that I spoke to, Julian had foreseen that there would be times when his accountability to his employer might threaten his ability or desire to do the right thing. Therefore:

> I very deliberately, during my late 30s and early 40s, lived modestly and saved and invested my salary in order to have what I think in the private sector is – somewhat inelegantly – called 'fuck you money' … I have always, from my early 40s, been in a position where I could

> walk away if I had to. And there have been times over the years when, if I had not had fuck you money, I would not have had the courage I've had.

The coercive force of corporate accountability had taken a great deal of work for him to overcome. His moral reasoning against corporate accountability relied on his professional ethics. Aware that professional ethics would be difficult to hold to if his line manager had the ability to cut his professional contract, Julian spent years building a protective wall of savings around his professional ethics. Unlike Betty, Julian's mortgage did not place such restrictive limits on how he translated his moral reasoning to practical actions and public discourse, but only because he had put time and effort into protecting his moral reasoning.[12]

Some of my other interlocutors found other ways of protecting themselves and their consciences. Olga, the nurse who organized the public meeting in Bolton, was dismissed from her role as a senior nurse in a mental health trust in 2007. She felt she was sacked as a result of her open criticism of the cuts being made at the time. I also spoke to an administrator in cancer care, Nancy, who had been suspended in the early 2000s due to her criticism of her manager's plans to change the pay structure within the trust. Both Olga and Nancy were union activists, seeking protection and strength in numbers, through collective action.

They both developed counter-arguments to their managers' plans. Olga's reasoning brought together moral arguments regarding worsening care for patients with self-interested arguments regarding mental health practitioners' terms and conditions of work. In Nancy's case, she was also criticizing a plan that would have had a deleterious effect on staff terms and conditions. In the union, one more accountability relationship was added, since Olga and Nancy were accountable to fellow employees. For Olga and Nancy, as holders of positions in their unions, they had a responsibility to contest changes that would have a negative effect on pay and work conditions. That is, Olga and Nancy were allied with other members of their respective unions. Their senses of responsibility were the basis of their reasoning, leading them to oppose more senior managers.

But both Olga and Nancy were heartened to see that other union members also felt accountable to them, as evidenced by these other employees taking action to protest their dismissals. It was the collective organization of the union that insulated them from corporate accountability. That is, whereas Julian had relied on his savings to have the courage to follow his professional ethics rather than corporate coercion, Olga and Nancy relied on the workplace bargaining power of the union to have the courage to follow reasoning that fulfilled their union responsibilities.[13]

Accountability, responsibility, obligation and alliance

In E.P. Thompson's (1991a) original description of moral economies, a disparate group of peasants, artisans and other workers came to see themselves as unified insofar as their ability to feed themselves and survive was threatened by changes in the economy. They petitioned the people they considered to be orchestrating the changes as well as people who were not in charge, but who were easily reachable, such as the sellers of bread, arguing that the 'patrician rulers' (1991a: 6) were foregoing the obligation they had previously held to ensure that everyone could at least subsist. Responsibility and obligation were moral concepts used discursively to contest changes in economic structures. Importantly, the use of these moral concepts aided certain groups of people – workers and peasants – to consider the ways in which they could form alliances with one another, while also leading them to consider other groups as moral antagonists. Emerging industrialists and politicians that led the arguments for the Corn Laws were petitioned along with the sellers of bread who were seen to be benefiting from higher prices.

In this chapter, I began by tracing how responsibility and accountability were redefined in the neoliberal era. In state organizations run under the auspices of NPM, accountability as audit functioned simultaneously as a means of working on the self in the crafting of the neoliberal subject, as well as a rationale for reducing and/or privatizing the services offered by the state.

Having recounted the history of neoliberal accountability, I described the various different ways I encountered people speaking of and using accountability in the moral economy of NHS transformation in Greater Manchester. Activists did not completely overhaul histories of ideas, nor did they pluck ideal concepts from the air. They worked with the social material available to them, as in Chapter 3 when they adapted their arguments to fit the NPM mantra of 'what matters is what works'. Activists contested changes to social and economic infrastructure by conceptualizing state structures as means of fulfilling moral obligations.

The responsibility envisaged by activists was a collective responsibility for members of society to take care for one another. The example described in Chapter 1 carried force because it was an existing structure that upheld this obligation. It was this obligation and the connected structure that they argued was being placed at risk.

Activists understood that certain actors at NHS England and in central government were most responsible for NHS changes. But they had no relation with those actors. Therefore, it was more local actors – the managers and politicians with whom they had relations – that they attempted to hold *accountable*. In putting their appeals to people like Theo, Brian and Betty, two social processes became apparent. First, activists became conscious of whom they were allying themselves with. They were arguing that the state was failing to meet its obligations to the whole public – all potential users of the NHS – rather than a specific interest group. Second, they forced Theo, Brian, Betty or whomsoever they attempted to hold accountable to position themselves on one of two sides: either on the side of activists and the general public, or the moral antagonist, the Tory government that was attempting to redraft the responsibilities of the state.

Conclusion

Activists mobilized moral arguments in their political action, attempting to hold someone accountable for organizational reforms that they considered to be wrong. The bureaucrats administering reforms evaded engagement with such arguments, citing the simple reality of constrained budgets. The managers had to balance the books.

But in interviews, the moral discourse of managers demonstrated that the disciplinary technologies of audit were not *quite* enough to enforce willing compliance. Their ethical imagination was not entirely enclosed, their openness to debate was not entirely foreclosed. Ideological closure was not wholly achieved. Audit could not eliminate contingency on its own. For Betty, the coercive pressure exerted through corporate accountability was required to enforce neoliberal transformation. It was the upwards accountability from periphery to centre, from locality to London, from trusts and CCGs to NHS England and central government, that stood out above other accountabilities and gave order to the mess. Central government was able to take advantage of a line of accountability from local managers and politicians all the way upwards to NHS England and the Department of Health and Social Care in Westminster that cut through all the other competing accountabilities, giving it the appearance of being inescapable.

Describing bureaucrats' justifications of their choices as ideological closure illuminates *how* they formed moral arguments in favour of service retrenchment: they were constrained by the reality of less money. This chapter goes further by explaining *why* they did. They were coerced under a previously scarcely examined rubric of neoliberal accountability: corporate accountability to one's employer. Rather than Muehlebach's (2012) moral neoliberal self, I have described the line managed neoliberal bureaucrat, her morality constrained within the menacing confines of the terms of her employment. If ever her moral reasoning suggested the capacity to build links and alliances with activists and the wider public, she was pressured such that her loyalty had to remain to the upwards accountability to the centre. Olga lost her job, Nancy was suspended, Betty simply *felt* the pressure. But Julian, Olga and Nancy all demonstrated that ideological closure did have cracks; alternatives were possible. It was possible for their moral reasoning to inform which side of the political battle they chose to place themselves on.

5

NHS Activism, Socialism and the Labour Party

In August 2018, I interviewed a Labour Party councillor, Maxine, in one of Greater Manchester's ten boroughs. It was a sunny day, and we sat outside a café in her district. She was the Executive Member for Social Care in her council cabinet and was in a position to describe local plans to change the NHS and social care. She spoke with passion about what they aimed to improve, but also qualified her statements with some reservations regarding the difficulties, particularly the lack of funds. A stereotype of slick disingenuity had informed my perception of some other politicians whom I interviewed. In contrast, I felt that Maxine was being honest about the kinds of problems that may derail the Labour-led council's goals. It felt to me as if she trusted me enough to be open about where the council might fail, rather than simply making false promises, like the managers described in Chapter 4.

Over the course of fieldwork, I had noticed that socialism was a recurring subject not just within NHS activism, but also within the Labour Party, as well as the wider sphere of political reporting and commentary. I had taken to asking people about whether they described themselves as socialists, and about what socialism meant to them. When I asked Maxine if she considered herself to be a socialist, it felt to me that the feeling of mutual trust suddenly evaporated. Up until that point, she had asked me very few questions. But then she began to probe about what *I* thought about my questions, what *my* motivations were, where my work would be published. To summarize, my use of the word 'socialist' appeared to make her suspicious.

Regarding socialism, she answered yes, but added a qualification, saying that she was a '*democratic* socialist', before saying that, actually, she did not want to be labelled. (She was not the first person to add this qualifier, 'democratic', when I asked interviewees if they considered themselves to be socialists. Many of the politicians had, and a few activists had.) She said that she wasn't sure what twenty-first-century socialism was, and then speculated:

> I think it's about good values ... I think it's about kindness, compassion, equality, fairness, accessibility, all those things. And I think you can do that as a good and decent person without having the label of a 'socialist' on you ... I'm a Labour Party member and I'm a Labour Party councillor and I have Labour Party values. And that is what I do, and it's about trying to get the best outcomes for the people that I represent across [her constituency]. And just generally being a good person, driving policy, changing policy for the best outcomes for people. Because that's what we're supposed to do in government, make things better for people.

In short, being a socialist, a Labour party member and a good person were synonymous for her.

Finally, she revealed what had irked her about the question: 'I think there's lots of sloganeering about what [socialism] is. And it feeds into the narrative: you're either for Corbyn or you're not for Corbyn. And I don't want to play that game frankly.' She was referring to something that I had already noticed among my interlocutors. NHS activists often referred to the people with whom they were in battle as 'not socialists', or 'not true socialists'. Maxine felt that the word 'socialist' had become a shorthand way of referring to the people on one side of a battle that was obscuring and interacting with the battles discussed in previous chapters. This other battle was between people who supported the leader of the Labour Party, Jeremy Corbyn, and people who opposed his leadership. Her point was that Corbyn's supporters referred to his detractors – or people they perceived as his detractors – as 'not socialist'. Many media commentators, Labour Party activists and members, including some of the people I was doing research with, considered this battle as one between 'left' and 'right' within the party. However, it was not always clear what left and right meant, who was on each side or why. Moreover, the battle over Corbyn's leadership was getting in the way of battles that Maxine deemed more immediately important: 'changing policy for the best outcomes for people'. What matters is what works.

Reflecting on the deployment of these signifiers – left, right, socialist – will be useful to further develop the story of whether and how groups were forming on the basis of a shared ethical vision. The previous two chapters demonstrated how cleavages and alliances took shape between the groups battling over the structure of the NHS, based on ethical judgements of the state and the state's obligations, in combination with direct coercion within bureaucratic power structures. This chapter places the story of NHS activism within the broader context of UK politics by relating my findings to the battles between left and right – 'socialists' and 'Blairites' – in the Labour Party.

The organizations I spent time with were deeply invested in the realignment of the Labour Party, especially the Socialist Health Association

(SHA), which was affiliated to it. Even the unaffiliated Dunning KONP and Greater Manchester KONP members were thinking through how to engage with the party and the ways in which it was changing. I follow how socialism was mobilized in the formation of alliances, how and to what kinds of ends. More precisely, how did a putative class politics – coalition-building within the party of labour – falter as it became entangled with moralized evaluations of persons?

The structure of the chapter is as follows: first, I briefly outline the recent history of the Labour Party. In this section, I combine literature from the anthropology of Britain with British and American socialist critique to describe how, until the ascent of Corbyn, Labour had become a party that had been transformed from the party of the working classes to a party that represented the interests of the professional-managerial class. I examine some of the literature on the professional-managerial class to set the scene for the difficulties and compromises faced by NHS activists. I then move on to explain the dilemmas experienced by Dunning KONP and Greater Manchester KONP with regard to whether and how to engage with the Labour Party. Next I explain how their dilemmas were analogous to much of the New Left's critique. Through the 1960s and 1970s, a changing but coherent critique emerged from a group of scholar-activists that came to be known as the New Left. They argued that, in fact, the Labour Party was *not* socialist, even if there were socialists in it. It was a party that was committed to improvement of capitalist structures through a parliamentary route that could never result in socialist transformation. The New Left critique acknowledged the sense that socialists had of the leadership repeatedly *betraying* socialist goals, but demoralized that betrayal by giving it a structural explanation. In the final section, I give a thick description of the tactics of organizing in the overlapping SHA and Labour Party. In this section, I demonstrate how suspicion and potential betrayal infected NHS activism, such that critiques of state structures often overlapped and interacted with evaluations of the ethics of individuals. Thus potential alliances were fractured before they had a chance to effect progressive change.

The Labour Party and the professional-managerial class

Jeremy Corbyn was elected leader of the Labour Party in 2015. Although he had been an MP since 1983, he had never held a cabinet post, and was not expected to win (Bale, 2016).[1] Successive leaders from 1983 onwards had explicitly sought to reposition the party to a political space often denoted as 'the centre'. Most notably, Tony Blair, leader from 1994 to 2007, had spearheaded New Labour, rejecting the seemingly tired 'shibboleths' of socialism, and the labels of left and right, instead focusing on the divisions between the politics of the past and the future (Robinson, 2017). Those shibboleths included Clause 4, a commitment in the party's constitution to campaign for the state to own the means of production in key industries. Clause 4 was replaced by a commitment to '*democratic* socialism' (my emphasis), emblazoned on the membership card even as the word, 'socialist' was omitted from any manifestos until 2017. The new politics, inspired by Giddens (1994; 1998) and the Third Way, sought not to curb markets, but to make use of them, following a logic of 'what matters is what works', closely linked to New Professional Management (NPM), as explored in previous chapters.

Blair's realignment of the party contributed to three successive election victories. Following his handover to Gordon Brown in 2007, the global financial crash hit in 2008. Labour then lost two successive elections, in 2010 under Gordon Brown's leadership and 2015 under Ed Miliband's.[2] Corbyn's victory in the subsequent leadership election suggested to many that the party may realign itself again, returning to a more 'socialist' position.

Anthropologists of Britain have largely studied not the politicians of the Labour Party, but how they have been perceived by citizens. Katherine Smith (2012) and Gillian Evans (2017) have described how working-class people[3] perceived changes in the Labour Party such that they felt betrayed by it. Insa Koch (2017) has documented how less wealthy people that in the past saw the Labour Party as the party that represented their interests, increasingly felt that no party represented them. Therefore, they rejected party politics *tout court*. The people whose interests were represented were 'people on high money' (Balthazar, 2017: 221). The social group so described was perceived to include not just financiers, rentiers and capitalists, not just the super-rich, but also the bureaucrats, managers and professionals that ran the state in a way that no longer protected working class and unemployed people, who instead experienced state interventions as 'punitive' (Koch, 2017: 228).

In his analysis of Labour's 2019 election defeat, Graeber (2020) wrote that in the 1990s, the party's pivot towards 'the center' was in essence a pivot towards representing the interests of the 'professional-managerial class'. This was not the first time Graeber had discussed the professional-managerial class (2014), nor the first time it had been associated with the international social democratic parties of the 1990s and 2000s (Press and Ehrenreich, 2019; Winant, 2019). The term originated with Barbara and John Ehrenreich (1977: 13), members of the American New Left who defined the professional-managerial class as 'salaried mental workers who do not own the means of production and whose major function in the social division of labor may be described broadly as the reproduction of capitalist culture and capitalist class relations'. The Ehrenreichs lamented how members of the professional-managerial class related to the working classes with contempt and paternalism, thus inhibiting potential alliances. Moreover, as a freestanding class, the professional-managerial class inhibited progress towards more egalitarian ways of structuring the state and society, since its aim was neither to overhaul capitalism nor to democratize workplaces and governments, but to, at best, improve state and capitalist structures through more efficient planning and social control. At worst, their role was to generate and enforce consent for – or acquiescence with – the prevailing economic system (Evans, 2023).

Over the years the meaning of the term changed, and in recent years it has become very common in socialist debates, in which the class is commonly referred to by the acronym, PMC.[4] As Winant (2019), an academic historian who also writes in left-leaning magazines, remarks:

> Spend time in the forums of socialists who've long been loyal to Sanders and critical of 'identity politics' – Jacobin readers, say, or in the listeners of Chapo Trap House – and you'll see 'PMC' everywhere, a sociological designation turned into an epithet and hurled like a missile.

Press (Press and Ehrenreich, 2019), another author in some of the same magazines as Winant, notes, 'the term has become a shorthand to point out that the interests of, say, pundits, or wealthier Democratic primary voters, aren't identical to those of working-class people'. Press describes the shift in the US's Democratic Party in the 1990s and 2000s in terms similar to Graeber's critique of the UK Labour Party. That is, its policy positions and rhetoric had changed to favour the interests of the PMC.

Winant (2019) describes how 'socialists' were seeking to realign the party in a way that would genuinely challenge neoliberal politics. Those who resisted this socialist challenge were now described as the PMC, with the term no longer describing *all* professionals and managers, since this social group no longer had the kinds of security of income and privilege that they once had. In the neoliberal era, especially after the global financial crash, they were a 'downwardly mobile' group experiencing real terms wage stagnation and precarity. As such, the current economic system was no longer working in their favour. But the Democratic Party continued to favour the interests of those professionals and managers whose wealth, assets and income had remained secure. In this new context the PMC was a battle cry and an insult used by socialists in the Democratic Party to denote the 'familiar enemies' who were still protected by the current economic order, 'the ones who made it, for whom good luck or preexisting advantages paid off, and who maintained their ultimate loyalty to the existing order.'

In this chapter, I will make comparisons between the PMC so described and the managers and politicians involved in the battles that have been portrayed in previous chapters. Ehrenreich (Press and Ehrenreich, 2019) has stated that she finds the recent usage of the term fascinating. But she worries that the transformation of the term is symptomatic of a problem with the contemporary left, of focusing too much on electoral politics rather than the development of alliances and the production of new, more egalitarian and democratic forms of decision-making. As we will see, her worries share some similarities with the British New Left critique of the Labour Party. I will focus on how such potential coalitions are sometimes being undermined within NHS activism rather than following Winant's (2019) advice: 'the point is not to abandon the PMC, but to turn it against its masters'.

Thus I seek to reinject the 'knots and potential entanglements' anthropologist Jane Cowan (2014: 95) referred to in political battles. In her critique of Graeber's (2014) account of the PMC, Cowan was referring to the messiness inherent in political battles. As people *try* to build alliances, their engagements overlap with strategizing influenced by other factors. In this chapter, those other factors will include moralized evaluations of familiar enemies. By 'moralized evaluations' I refer to how interpersonal interactions between potential allies are influenced by strategic considerations, in which victory over some sort of electoral opponent is paramount. And those strategic considerations interact with judgements of an individual's character. I demonstrate how perceptions and moral judgements of people interact with perceptions of 'sides' in a political battle that coalesced around interpretations of left and right, good socialists and not socialists.

Greater Manchester KONP – the Labour Party is the only game in town

Dunning KONP and Greater Manchester KONP are both affiliated to the national organization, KONP. All three organizations explicitly state that they are not affiliated to any political parties. Therefore, I found it remarkable just how much we talked about the Labour Party within both Dunning KONP and Greater Manchester KONP. The party came up at every formal meeting, and many, if not most, informal conversations. Some of these conversations were to be expected; after all, we had Labour-led or Labour majority councils in all of Greater Manchester's boroughs, and a Labour Party Mayor. However, it was often the national Labour Party that we were talking about, rather than the local Labour Party.

As described in Chapters 1 and 3, several of the most active members of Greater Manchester KONP were now retired, but had been active in their unions throughout their careers and thus considered that they had been NHS activists since the 1980s. They agreed that following the election of Corbyn, now was an interesting time for the Labour Party, an appropriate time to engage with it. However, they differed on their views on how – and how much – to engage.

Catherine, a retired health promotion worker, mentioned in one Greater Manchester KONP meeting that she had decided to 'hold my nose and join the Labour Party'. When I had lunch with her, Ruth and Debbie, I asked her why she had to hold her nose. She told me that she knew there would be people in the Labour Party who held completely opposite views to her on what the NHS should look like and how it should be changed. That is, there were people in the Labour Party that she did not consider to be socialists.

Catherine gave the example of a Labour Party member who used to be an MP, Neil Turner. She told me that Turner was on the board of WWL Solutions, the subsidiary company to which Wrightington, Wigan and Leigh NHS Foundation Trust was planning to transfer many of its staff, as described in Chapter 3. The trust had proposed that large groups of non-clinical staff would be transferred to WWL Solutions. The transfer meant that they would no longer be employed by the NHS, thus removing them from national NHS staff collective pay bargaining. The involvement of a Labour politician in the company demonstrated for Catherine that there were people in Labour who went beyond passive toleration or rhetorical support of privatization. They actively participated in privatizing parts of the NHS and thus could not be described as socialists.

Ruth, also a retired health promotion worker, was more forthright than simply describing such people as not socialist. She described them as 'Blairites', a term that has become an insult in the battles within the Labour Party, with Blair serving as a figurehead of the period in which Labour deviated from socialism.[5] Ruth had no interest in joining the Labour Party, since she felt that it remained dominated and run by Blairites, even with a socialist as nominal leader. But she agreed that now was a good time to engage with it, because it was 'the only game in town', 'the only large-scale expression of working-class demands'. Since she understood Corbyn to be a socialist, Corbyn's victory suggested to her that this was a good time to intervene and strengthen those demands. She wanted to stimulate discussions about the NHS within the Labour Party, which she felt was not openly discussing what had happened and what was going on in the NHS. Her particular problem was the lack of discussion of the Labour Party's own contribution to privatization. She hoped that if she and other KONP members could stimulate such a discussion, then Labour members might see how Labour politicians themselves had contributed to undermining the NHS and its values. Thus, these politicians would be exposed as 'right wing' or 'Blairite', and KONP would have made a positive contribution to the battle between left and right in the Labour Party.

But Ruth predicted that Corbyn would ultimately fail to transform the Labour Party into a socialist party. As she put it, 'I don't think that the Corbyn project will work. In the long-term I think it'll be defeated. And therefore, I want independent socialist groups, [including] KONP … to maintain themselves independent of the Labour Party, but taking … what is going on in the Labour Party very seriously.' Labour was important because of its size and its influence, but she felt that converting the party itself into an effective instrument for socialist transformation was a project doomed to failure. However, she argued that it could still be used to build a wider movement that could eventually effect socialist goals.[6]

Ruth and Catherine combined short-term goals of changing or influencing Labour politicians with longer-term goals of raising an awareness among Labour members that Labour politicians do not always serve the interests of working people or Labour members. Thus we see a mixture of ambivalence ('hold my nose'), compromise (join or engage anyway because it is 'the only game in town') and tactical manoeuvring to build on the predicted inevitability of defeat. In Ruth's case, her consideration of advancing towards a good society incorporated a sense that the struggle to get there had to be undertaken by working people themselves. Therefore, the role of socialist activists had to be to find ways to build the working class's consciousness of who had acted in its interests, and who had not. That is, the Labour Party was important due to being the party with the most members, particularly working-class members, but the task of true socialists was to reveal to those members that there were people working against their interests even within the Labour Party. The most important battle was not just between Labour and other parties, but between socialists and not socialists. Socialism had to be separated from the Labour Party, since not everyone in the Labour Party was a true socialist, working towards a vision of a better society with which Ruth and Catherine agreed. The NHS was useful for using as a simple marker for who was or was not a socialist. If you apologized for – or actively participated in – privatization in the NHS, then you could not possibly be a socialist.

Ruth's tactical manoeuvring sought to clarify exactly what kinds of alliances had been enshrined within and by the 'broad church'[7] Labour Party. If the people with greatest influence over the Labour Party's actions were in favour of privatization, then they were not acting in the interests of working-class people. Ruth wanted members to realize that a stratum of Labour politicians – Ruth did not call them a PMC, but the epithet would fit – had formed an alliance with a capitalist class that hitched the party to the interests of capital. In short, Ruth felt that there was strategic value in stoking conflict in the party, to build a consciousness among members of who was on their side, and who was not. The sides concretized around two words: socialist and Blairite.

Dunning KONP – the most important thing is getting a Labour government

Whereas Ruth was actively trying to stoke conflict within the Labour Party, Dunning KONP members were more circumspect regarding the short-term consequences of such conflict, particularly for winning elections. At Dunning KONP meetings, they debated different ways to engage with Labour locally. They were conscious that the Labour-led council was pushing through reforms with which they disagreed, but wary of shouting too loudly about their disagreements, for fear of increasing the probability of the Tories or Liberal Democrats winning seats in future elections and pushing through reforms that were even worse.

Esther and her husband, Dean, were at the heart of the debates in Dunning KONP. They were among the people who had joined after that first meeting in 2012, after hearing Galen and Iris speak about the Health and Social Care Act. Esther had joined Labour in 2004, but had been inspired by Corbyn recently, becoming more active in her branch, being elected vice-chair of her CLP (Constituency Labour Party[8]) and joining the pro-Corbyn pressure group, Momentum.[9] She told me that she wanted Dunning KONP to influence Dunning council, which was led by Labour, but she deemed that they should place a limit on how much to publicly criticize the Labour Party. She calculated that the best way to serve Dunning KONP's aims – which she saw as stopping cuts and privatization in the NHS – was to get a Labour national government as soon as possible. Therefore, she argued that Dunning KONP should always consider whether a proposed action would contribute to getting Labour back into power or hinder that goal. If the latter, then they should not do it:

> That is our only hope, to get a Labour government. And that is why I've had so much of a problem with the antagonism of Dunning Council. Because I believe success filters, you know, and if we're criticizing Dunning Council I'm worried that Labour won't be elected again. Labour will be seen as a failure locally, and that will be mirrored in the national elections … The only way we're going to save the NHS is with a Labour government. We've got to get these Tories out.

Her enthusiasm for Labour was not universally shared within Dunning KONP. Nor was her explicit linkage of Dunning KONP's aims to a Labour government. Disagreements regarding how to discuss Labour and its actions in local government bubbled to the surface in the run-up to the general election in 2017. This was just before I started fieldwork but several of my interviewees told me about it. Esther and Dean argued that Dunning KONP should campaign for Labour. Others agreed with the premise that Labour were the best option, but also wanted to preserve Dunning KONP's independence from any party-political alliance. The chair of Dunning KONP, Wes, described its most important role as 'speaking truth to power'. He thought that the ability to perform this role would be undermined by supporting a particular party, as the public would then see Dunning KONP as simply that party's 'mouthpiece'. Danny, himself a councillor, felt that if Dunning KONP did not criticize the Labour council's NHS policies then nobody else would have the expertise or knowledge to do so. (Danny was the only Labour councillor in Dunning who opposed the council's plans for the NHS.)

Eventually, the group decided not to support Labour. But it did participate in campaigning, instead advising the public not to vote Tory. They concluded that they could preserve their independence from any one political party while still criticizing the governing party. In summary, they argued that a vote for the Tories was a vote *against* the NHS, evidenced by the cuts forced on NHS trusts and local governments. They found little success with this strategy. People shouted at them on the street, and the areas where they campaigned did return Tory MPs. Moreover, as a result of his disagreement with the strategic decision not to explicitly support Labour, Dean stopped attending Dunning KONP meetings. Esther continued to attend, but voiced some frustration, particularly with Wes.

When the 2018 *local* elections came up during my fieldwork, the stakes were different. Even Esther and Dean agreed that there were significant parts of the Labour-led council's plans which Dunning KONP should criticize. However, Labour remained a better option than the other parties. As Iris put it, 'One bucket of sick is better than two buckets of sick.' Following their experience at the 2017 general election, this time they decided not to participate at all. Instead, they remained 'quiet' in the preceding month, so as not to reduce the Labour vote. They did not organize any pamphleting, write any letters or attend any council, Clinical Commissioning Group (CCG) or trust meetings to ask difficult questions. Labour gained one additional seat and lost none.

In essence, they formed a tacit alliance with the local Labour Party (although I do not know if any Labour politicians were actually aware of their purposeful inactivity), in recognition of their belief that Labour represented 'one bucket of sick' rather than two. That is, Dunning KONP members objected to Labour's actions, but felt unable to criticize them since such criticism would increase the probability of getting 'two buckets of sick'.

Around the same time, Danny informed the group that senior councillors were considering whether to change the structure of cabinet meetings.[10] Danny had heard from some colleagues that the cabinet were considering removing the ability to submit and ask questions of cabinet members. Everyone in Dunning KONP agreed that councillors must have made this decision in response to Dunning KONP asking difficult questions.

Up until this point, most of them had interpreted the councillors' irritation as evidence that their strategy of asking questions was *working*. Wes said to me during an interview just before Danny's news, 'They don't really like us very much. But for me that's a positive thing because at least it means we're annoying them.' If the councillors were annoyed, they knew they were being watched, and could not 'get away with' secretive or underhand actions that were not in the public's interest. This formed part of what the group referred to as holding councillors to account. Here I focus on the sentiment, widely shared in Dunning KONP, that the exasperation of councillors (of which they also had much more evidence) suggested that Dunning KONP were on the right course. Esther was one of the few who disagreed, arguing that councillors, infuriated by incessant questions and unrealistic demands, no longer took Dunning KONP seriously. Therefore, their criticisms were not having an influence on local government, which Esther took as further ballast for her primary argument that Dunning KONP should concentrate on campaigning for a national Labour government.

At a meeting in February 2018, Danny told the group that the council were discussing whether to restrict questions. Their first response was anger. Most of the group saw the potential loss of this avenue of critique as an undemocratic exercise of power by the cabinet. Iris, bristling and gesticulating, said, 'they make you go from calm to apoplectic in three seconds … It's 1984 playing out before our eyes … They are judge and jury.' Although others were less effusive, most shared her displeasure.

However, there was less agreement over how to proceed. Wes had said to me in our interview that Dunning KONP's most important aim was speaking truth to power, through open and unlimited critique. But now he suggested that Dunning KONP should consider tempering their critique in order to keep this avenue of communication open. He replied to Iris, 'I think you are exaggerating a bit … It's a game and you need to play the game.' Later, he added, 'You don't win a chess game by throwing the board off the table.' Another member guffawed, 'We need a new board'. Wes replied, 'It's not going to happen … We don't want to lose this avenue'.

Here we see the group working out strategies of compromise in order to remain engaged with local governmental politics. Throughout this section, we have seen ambivalence towards the Labour Party. On the one hand, Dunning KONP considers that it is compelled to engage with it as it is the ruling party locally, and the *only* party nationally that can win a general election and reverse cuts and privatization. On the other hand, Dunning KONP found itself frustrated by their lack of success in influencing politicians, and by the forms of engagement allowed by the parliamentary system. They were wary of the kinds of compromises that they felt they were being forced into, and yet saw no other options available to them. Allying themselves with the Labour Party necessarily affected what they considered possible and achievable.

The New Left critique – Labour, a party with socialists in it

From the late 1950s onwards, a group of scholars emerged that have become known as the New Left. 1968 is commonly seen as a breaking point between older members of this group, such as E.P. Thompson, and newer members, such as Perry Anderson and Tom Nairn (Davis, 2003). The New Left brought a new strain of Marxism to British academia, including a critique of the Labour Party. Their basic thesis was that although there were socialists in the Labour Party, the party could not itself be described as a socialist party because it was an obstacle to the transformation of society from capitalism to socialism. In this section, I briefly outline why New Left intellectuals found the party problematic, before comparing their dilemmas to those of NHS activists.

Ralph Miliband (2009 [1961]) argued that since the Labour Party was hitched to an inherently non-democratic and conservative first-past-the-post parliamentary system, its transformative potential was severely limited. Anderson (1964) and Nairn (1964a; 1964b) elaborated further on the history of class conflict in England and the UK, making comparisons with other European countries. Whereas the revolutions of 1789 to 1848 had decisively installed the bourgeoisie as the ruling class in mainland Europe, the bourgeoisie of England had formed more of a coalition with the aristocracy, taking on some of their airs and graces rather than chopping off their heads.

In addition to this incomplete class overthrow, England grew away from its European counterparts. Whereas working class parties in mainland Europe had intellectuals that could theorize a counter-hegemonic ideology – where the accepted hegemony was some version of liberal capitalism – the Labour Party's intellectuals remained geographically insular (except in their self-conceptualization as masters of the empire), drawing on Bentham and Malthus rather than Marx and Engels (Davis, 2003). The Labour Party drew its intellectual inspiration from Fabian empiricism and reformism rather than a revolutionary, emancipatory imagination. Anderson wrote that 'a supine bourgeoisie produced a supine proletariat' (1964).

Within the New Left, there were disagreements and changes of opinion over whether the Labour Party would *always* remain an obstacle to socialist transformation, and whether it could or should be used as a vehicle of socialist progress. Some members of the group, such as Ralph Miliband, did become involved with the party (holding his nose like Catherine), only to find themselves frustrated by parliamentary politics and ultimately deciding that Labour was irredeemable (Newman, 2003). But even those who never dabbled in Labour politics could not find their way around the problem that Labour was the party with the most working-class members,[11] and to which the working classes felt the greatest affiliation. In a two-party parliamentary system that hindered the development of other parties, the New Left ultimately suffered a 'failure of nerve' (Davis, 2003: 42). They criticized the party as doomed to inevitable defeat in its advancement of socialist progress, and yet did not – could not – find or create an alternative. In summary, Labour was the only game in town.

The Nairn-Anderson theses are decades old but remain influential (Hannah, 2018; Finn, 2019). Perry Anderson (2020) has recently asserted that its arguments have held up well. Bassett (2019) has argued that Corbyn's Labour fell foul of the same weaknesses of labourism[12] decried by the New Left. But there were critiques of the Nairn-Anderson theses from within the New Left. E.P. Thompson felt that the Nairn-Anderson thesis lacked depth. In Thompson's estimation, their abstract analysis did not take stock of the empirical material available, which revealed the 'Peculiarities of the English' (1965: 311). Thompson argued that Anderson and Nairn's analysis started from a hidden ideal type against which to compare labourism, thus leading them to insist that socialism had to be Marxist and revolutionary. Therefore, since labourism lacked a robust Marxist basis, Anderson and Nairn were able to dismiss English radicalism as non-socialist, without recourse to further examination.[13]

As well, Nairn and Anderson could not describe what it felt like to be an English socialist or Labour member. A sense of betrayal was often mentioned (and still is by Labour members who consider themselves to be on the left (Hannah, 2018)), but rather than being explored and explained, it was explained *away* as the inevitable result of labourism:

> The Milibandian thesis was never that an inherently socialist working class was periodically betrayed by Labour Party moderation. It was rather that the possibility of creating such a radicalized class has been blocked by, among other things, the presence of a party committed to Labourism rather than socialism, and the periodic leftwards shift in rhetoric made by the Labour Party whenever working-class militancy intensified … The whole thrust of the Milibandian argument on the working class and socialism was that the fusion between the two was one that had to be *created*, and that such a creation required clear and unambiguous political leadership of a kind that the Labour Party systematically declined to offer. (Coates and Panitch, 2003: 74–75, emphasis in original)

For the New Left, socialists were not betrayed by non-socialists. Socialism was blocked by labourism, by the fact of the Labour Party's existence as either Her Majesty's Government or Her Majesty's Most Loyal Opposition and its consequent adherence to the rules of British parliamentary democracy. We saw varying levels of recognition of this problem among my research participants in the previous sections of this chapter. Dunning KONP's disagreements over how to interact with the Labour Party gave us an example of the kinds of compromises that result from engagement with the parliamentary system. Calculations regarding what was politically possible led to reconsideration of what was ethically desirable. Even when everyone in

Dunning KONP shared the same goal of criticizing and stopping cuts and privatization in the NHS, they could not agree on how to go about doing so. And they ended up having to temper their critique in order to reduce conflict with Labour politicians, and thus continue to have a voice within the local government's cabinet.

On the other hand, Greater Manchester KONP were more detached from the 'ultimate' goal of maintaining power for Labour in local government or gaining power for Labour in national government. Instead they actively encouraged difficult questions within the Labour Party in order to achieve the longer-term goals of socialist transformation of the party itself, and the consciousness of working people associated with the party. But Ruth and Catherine did so by focusing on individuals who had betrayed the interests of the working classes, people who were not socialists, but Blairites.

In the next section I focus on the senses of betrayal and mutual suspicion that coalesced around the concept of socialism, with moralized evaluations of persons becoming intertwined with and inseparable from broader conceptualizations of how to realize the good society. These feelings took shape within battles for control of the party that were influenced by the adversarial, winner-takes-all nature of parliamentary politics. I follow how these parliamentary dynamics interacted with judgements of people, thus affecting how coalitions did or did not form.

The Socialist Health Association

The SHA was originally conceived by socialist doctors as the State Medical Services Association, after the First World War. These doctors believed that a socialized medical service – universal, free and served by full-time, state employed staff – was not only a noble goal, but could serve as a 'model for socialism' (Stewart, 1999: 1). But many members were frustrated by the isolation and lack of influence of the organization. Therefore, these members broke away and formed the Socialist Medical Association (SMA), which affiliated to the Labour Party. It was through Labour that the SMA sought to realize its aims.[14]

At the start of my fieldwork, both Ronny and Charles held important positions in the SHA. Both had been involved with the SHA for some time, and Charles was also involved with KONP. They were both able to help me a great deal with my fieldwork, signposting me towards other groups I was not previously aware of, and connecting me to other people. It was Ronny that sent round an email to his contacts that led to most of my interviews with NHS managers. He understood building networks with such bureaucrats to be a key part of his role as an SHA activist. Interestingly, this fraternizing with the proponents of the reforms campaigners opposed was also an important factor contributing to him being mistrusted by those activists. Ronny appeared to be on the side of the people with whom many other activists were in battle.

But the key factor in other activists' mistrust of Ronny was their belief that he was not a socialist. Often the members of Greater Manchester KONP and Dunning KONP that knew Ronny went further and described him as a Blairite. Mistrust of Ronny frequently extended to mistrust of the whole SHA. Some of my friends told me that the SHA was Ronny's 'fiefdom'. Even those who supported and trusted Ronny had a tendency to consider him as representative of the whole organization, as suggested by the supportive messages he received on social media after he lost his position. Many of them repeated the same words, 'You *are* the SHA'.[15]

One of the people whom I heard describing Ronny as a Blairite was Charles. Separately, Ronny told me that he knew Charles mistrusted him and that Charles thought he was a Blairite.[16] I saw evidence of this mistrust not just in our interviews, but also in meetings, in which Charles often made comments or jokes about their political disagreements. For example, at a meeting in November 2017, SHA members were discussing a document that had already been circulated around the members. One member wanted to change some of the words. Ronny objected to the change, initially on the grounds that it would denigrate the role of the voluntary sector in the NHS. Ronny then objected on the basis of organizational process, saying that the document had already been circulated a while ago, so it was not fair to suggest a change so late in the day. Both Ronny and the other member had raised their voices, so Charles had asked all members to behave in a 'comradely fashion'. A calmer discussion ensued and some resolution was reached whereby the working group would look at it again. In summing up, Charles mentioned that Ronny had been involved in writing the document. Ronny interrupted, 'No, I wasn't.' Charles replied, 'Oh, sorry. I thought you were.' Ronny said, 'No, I just took some words out.' Another member, Mandy, quipped, 'Not the right ones obviously.' Charles said, 'No, Mandy. The *left* ones.'

Charles described himself as a socialist. Others also described him as a socialist. I often heard activists who were aware of Charles's role in the SHA describe him as returning the SHA to being socialist, after a long period of non-socialism under the aegis of Ronny, the Blairite. We see here how activists' perceptions of the beliefs and actions of Ronny and Charles – with regard to advancing particular notions of what state medical services should look like – contributed to their moralized evaluations of the persons themselves. People who agreed with Charles's vision liked and trusted Charles, the socialist. He was a 'good' or 'true socialist'. (He was also congenial and affable; I was one of the many people who liked Charles.) But the same people who trusted Charles mistrusted and avoided Ronny, the Blairite. As Danny, the Dunning KONP member and councillor, put it to me during an interview, 'He's not really a socialist'. Most of the activists with whom I spent time preferred Charles to Ronny. Some of the managers and politicians with whom I spent time were closer to Ronny.

Labour Party conference speeches in favour of an SHA motion co-written by Charles[17] were widely shared and watched on social media, and the SHA saw a spike in membership after the conference. But the motion was probably not the only factor. A number of other socialist societies also saw spikes in membership around a similar time, such as the Labour Irish Society. Corbyn-supporting blogs and organizations such as Momentum had been encouraging Corbyn-supporting members – that is, the people who understood themselves to be the Labour left – to join socialist societies for some time, arguing that the Labour right had already done so. Momentum released a set of videos aiming to educate new Labour members about how the party works, with a view to helping them to wield influence within their local party organizations. A key reason for all of this activity was that socialist societies are able to elect delegates within CLPs. Although some long-standing members described such tactics as 'Trotskyist infiltration' or 'entryism', the people that I spoke to felt that the Labour right had a long history of using socialist societies (as well as unions) to 'pack the room' with delegates who would obstruct socialist, left-wing motions and policy.

The SHA's increase in membership was a national phenomenon. But it had significant ramifications in Manchester. Towards the end of 2017, Ronny began to talk about setting up a local branch of the SHA, in Greater Manchester. There had been one in the past, but some of the members had left and others had died, so the group had disintegrated. But now that membership was increasing, Ronny suggested that it might be a good time to set one up again. Ronny called a planning meeting in early 2018, and an inaugural Annual General Meeting (AGM) was held in March. Before the AGM, there was a drastic surge in membership which then became the focus of discussion and innuendo. Charles told me later that 198 people joined in Greater Manchester in the two months before the AGM. For context, the national membership had risen to 964 in March 2018, from 792 in 2017.[18]

I witnessed some of how this large increase in membership in Greater Manchester came about. In February 2018, I was added to a Facebook group of Labour members, many of whom I recognized as people who were generally supportive of Corbyn. Initially most people in the group were not sure why it had been created. The person who created the group, Jim, outlined its aims: 'Go to AGM – get delegates for CLPs – weaken the grip of establishment/right, while fighting for a free, publicly run and owned NHS'. The main point of this particular Facebook group was to organize people to join the SHA and attend the AGM in order to vote for other left (Corbyn-supporting) committee members and delegates to CLPs.

The group was interesting to me for the debate as to the purpose of the group itself, and the purpose of joining the SHA. Following Jim's statement above, one person suggested that the purpose of the group was to organize a slate of candidates for committee positions and CLP delegates who all supported Corbyn. Another person objected with regard to the purpose of joining the SHA, 'I hope we're all up for campaigning … rather than just delegates to CLPs. The second is important, but not as important as defending our NHS'. The first person replied, 'Absolutely. I'd hope that's a given for socialists.'

The discussion reveals how the two goals – campaigning against cuts and privatization in the NHS and taking control of the Labour Party – had become very difficult to separate from one another. Ronny and Charles both told me that they were worried about people joining the SHA purely for the latter goal who were not interested in the former. That is, people might be using the SHA as a vehicle in a party-political battle, albeit one still undergirded by an ethical vision of how the state and society should be structured. And both Ronny and Charles suspected the 'other side' more than their own. That is, Ronny was concerned regarding left-wing infiltration, and Charles was concerned about right-wing infiltration. They both suspected subversion of the SHA's rules. Their political concerns led them to suspect individuals of immoral behaviour. When the SHA was rejuvenated by new members who sought to organize themselves in order to wield more influence, presumably in order to be more effective in campaigning for what they saw as good and right, their actions were recast as morally suspect. Moreover, the new members themselves absorbed and reproduced these moralized evaluations of the other side, incorporating them into their strategies, and even the need to form sides in the first place.

Most of my experience was with the people who considered themselves to be on the left, who felt that they needed to organize *as* the left, the 'true socialists', in order to combat the right, who they felt had been well organized for years, and thus in the ascendancy. Ronny informed me that the right really *were* organizing to combat the left. The left grouping was at least partially correct in its suspicions. Ronny told me that one Manchester MP, a Corbyn critic, had been spooked by the amount of new members in the SHA. Since she was worried that these new members would be 'lefty, Momentum-y types' (as Ronny described them) who might be delegated to her CLP and wield influence against her, she led a campaign of recruiting her own supporters to the SHA. Ronny told me that the Greater Manchester branch's membership swelled from 80 in 2017 to more than 300 after the AGM in 2018.

Although the AGM itself passed without incident, the mutual suspicion between sides did sometimes bubble up to the surface, revealing the underlying tension. On the way back from the AGM, it occurred to me that a trade union liaison officer may be a useful position to add to the committee, to facilitate effective communication and education of NHS staff with regard to how cuts and privatization were affecting local services. I sent an email to the whole branch outlining my thoughts. A few people replied with supportive comments, before one person replied, 'I think someone could work in that area but I do not think it necessary or appropriate to keep on inventing extra officer positions … Inventing extra officer positions is now a tactic used by Momentum to take over committees.' A bitter exchange of emails ensued, in which I did not participate. Ronny eventually settled it by asking people not to make accusations of improper motives without evidence.

In the exchange, as with other email exchanges, it was clear that two sides formed around the lines explored in this chapter: left and right. The most obvious distinguishing characteristics between left and right were support for Corbyn and tolerance of private companies and voluntary sector organizations in the NHS. Those who perceived themselves as the left supported Corbyn and did not accept any role for private or voluntary organizations in the NHS. But this email exchange was about neither of those things; it was simply about committee positions in the SHA. And yet it *seemed* clear to me that those who supported my proposition were on the left, and those who suspected me (and/or Momentum) of simply inventing positions as a power play were on the right. The seeming clarity of my perceptions demonstrates how one consequence of the suspicion at play in these battles was that sides solidified and perceptions of the other crystallized. I thought I could predict the political views of the people who engaged in the discussion on the basis of which side they took.

Such accusations of foul play were commonplace, although I normally only heard Corbyn-supporting members voicing them in closed groups. (I was not party to the closed groups of the other side except through what Ronny told me.) Within the SHA, it was rare for the accusations to be made so openly. On the other hand, national media regularly reported on similar accusations in the national Labour Party, with Labour MPs accusing members of 'entryism', 'Trotskyist infiltration' or 'hard left takeovers'. It was easy for me to see the SHA as a microcosm of the national Labour Party, with two factions basing their strategizing on a conspiratorial imagination, a sense of a perceived other – either the left or the right – organizing in a way that placed one's own side at threat.

What was at stake was not just the strength of one's own side, but the realization of its ethical vision of how the political structures of the state should be organized. The only way to combat the other side's potential betrayal was to organize one's own side. And when the other side became aware of one side's organizing, they comprehended it as further evidence of conspiracy. Within the SHA, the end result, after the end of my fieldwork and Ronny's dismissal, was the suspension of the Greater Manchester branch by the national officers, who suspected that the aforementioned Manchester MP's recruitment campaign had breached organizational rules. When Charles spoke to me of his interpretation of the MP's actions, he said, 'Something's going to have to happen or these people are going to continue to exert unethical influence on the SHA'.

In pinning down these moralized perceptions of the other side, we begin to move away from the theoretical abstraction of the New Left critique of the Labour Party, instead exploring how the political trajectory of one socialist society – a microcosm of the party at large – played out in the nitty-gritty of everyday relations between two sides. Although *who* was on each side seemed very clear to most of the actors, with Ronny and Charles standing as emblematic of right and left respectively, *what* exactly each side represented was less clear to me. I make no attempt to explain away the sense of betrayal in the way that the New Left critique did. Instead I argue that a sense of potential betrayal is central to the perception of the other, and to the subsequent group formation.

Ronny initially felt that some of the seeming political fissures between him and Charles were simply due to poor or inadequate communication. In September 2017, Ronny told me, 'I don't disagree with [Charles] about very much'. Again, as with KONP members, one of the main points of divergence in their consideration of current and future NHS reforms was over privatization. Ronny was significantly less worried that current reforms would lead to privatization, as well as being less convinced that the use of independent sector organizations was a problem anyway. However, he did subscribe to the key principles of universality and comprehensiveness of a free service that should aim to provide equally excellent services for all.

As already mentioned, when I asked other Dunning KONP and Greater Manchester KONP members to elaborate on their mistrust of Ronny and the SHA, they described him as a Blairite who fraternized with the managers who were pushing through the reforms to which they objected. However, they also often related stories of interactions with him in which they portrayed him as rude, brusque or dismissive. For example, I heard several people describe having expressed worries regarding privatization to him. He would respond, 'Well, what has been privatized in your area?' People's responses here varied. Some people were unaware of specific services that had been privatized, some described non-clinical services that had been contracted out and others explained that their concern was actually regarding the potential for future privatization that had been opened by current reforms. Ronny interpreted these interactions as evidence that many 'KONP demonstrator type people' were 'not very knowledgeable … and quite a lot of them don't really know very much about what's actually happening. And I think that's a problem. And I'm not against those sorts of people, some of them are lovely, but I think the SHA is a lot more effective if we can produce people who do actually know what they're talking about. Not just saying "this is a load of shite"'.

Dunning KONP and Greater Manchester KONP members interpreted Ronny's tone as evidence of a lack of sympathy for left-wing views; he was not a socialist, he was a Blairite, and he was patronizing to boot. Their personal interactions with Ronny, his manner of speaking, his means of address, even his clothes, coloured and overlapped with evaluations of him as a person. These evaluations then contributed to decisions regarding how to interact with the political organization that many felt was inextricably linked to him. Moralized judgements of persons were impossible to separate from the ethics and politics of state healthcare and the political activism thereof. Decisions regarding who to form alliances with, who was on your side and who was on the other side, were shaped by the interplay between these evaluative fields: personal, ethical, political.

The impossibility of separating these fields was further demonstrated when Ronny lost his position in the SHA.[19] As far as I could understand from what Ronny and Charles told me, and the various official emails I received as a member, due process was followed by the organization. In fact, Ronny did not deny having done any of the things that the tribunal found that he had done. He only disputed the severity of the punishment – dismissal from the SHA – for those actions. But Ronny still interpreted the developments following his alleged breaches as a conspiracy against him, motivated by a perception that he was a Blairite, not a socialist.[20]

Two sides formed and solidified around these perceptions of what the other side was doing. These perceptions then contributed to strategizing in such a way that seemed to perpetuate the mistrustful circle. Although there appeared to be some symmetries to each side's organizing, each side construed the other as morally suspect, and their own organizing as necessary in the context of an overarching goal of overcoming the other side. The undergirding purpose of overcoming the other side was to realize an ethical vision of achieving a better, fairer society through an alternative structuring of the NHS to that proposed by current reforms. And much of what was happening in the SHA was also happening in the national Labour Party. After he told me about John's conspiracy theory, I suggested to Ronny that everyone seems to mistrust everyone. He agreed, telling me:

> Yes, I think you could say that. Well, it's like the Labour Party. I mean, that's the bit I don't like about the Labour Party and the SHA. Whereas in previous years people have managed to get on, now there's a great deal of suspicion and shouting at people because you're not in my gang, essentially.

The gangs he referred to were what I have been describing as sides in a political battle, where people on one side agree with one another on how to make progress towards a fairer society by means of changing state structures, using the Labour Party as a vehicle through which to do so. Although in previous chapters I have sketched some notions of how the NHS might serve as an icon of such a socialist society, here I stress that the formation of battle lines around the concepts of socialism, left and right often led to skating over what such a society might look like or how we might go about realizing it. Moralized evaluations of persons interacted with and sometimes replaced ethical reasoning with regard to state structures. The Blairites had to be overcome. They had to be overcome because they were not socialists. The Momentum-y types had to be overcome. They had to be overcome because they were Corbynite conspirators.

Conclusion

This chapter has tracked the alliances and coalitions built by NHS activists within and alongside the Labour Party. The first half of the chapter focused on Greater Manchester KONP and Dunning KONP, two organizations that considered themselves to be independent of party-political affiliation. Despite this supposed independence, they were ineffably hitched to the Labour Party, 'the only game in town', for the realization of socialist goals and the protection of the NHS as they saw it. I explored how their engagements with the party influenced their reasoning and practice. Aligning with the Labour party did not mean creating an unproblematic alliance with all people in the UK, nor even all working-class people.

Electoral victory for the parliamentary Labour party was a key concern not just for party members, but for all NHS activists. This concern led Dunning KONP members to make various compromises in order not to reduce the chances of Labour winning. But Greater Manchester KONP members took a different approach. Ruth predicted that neither Corbyn nor the party could succeed in effecting socialist goals. Therefore, she focused on revealing the class politics of the Labour Party to its own members. She wanted members to understand the Labour Party's role in tolerating or furthering privatization, which she understood as evidence that the party served the interests of the professional-managerial class. Ruth's analysis shared some similarities with anthropological writing on the Labour Party (Smith, 2012; Evans, 2017; Graeber, 2020), a key theme of which has been betrayal; Labour politicians had betrayed socialist goals and/or the working classes by allowing the NHS to be privatized. The people in control of the party had reshaped it in the interests of the PMC, allying themselves with capital rather than the residents of the UK, or the working classes.

The second half of the chapter followed the sense of betrayal or potential betrayal in the SHA; a socialist society affiliated to the Labour Party. I shone a light on intra-party relations at a moment when the ascent of Corbyn created a hope for many that the party might realign itself away from the interests of the PMC, towards the 'left', towards 'socialism'. These words and, especially, their supposed opposites, 'right' and 'Blairite', became sticky, opaque signifiers, insults to 'be hurled like a missile' (Winant, 2019) at opponents. The concept of 'socialism' became a shorthand in a political battle that sometimes short-circuited and perpetuated the battle. By 'short-circuit', I mean that a concern for how to overcome the opposite side in order to realize one's own side's vision sometimes led to an elision of discussion of what the other side's vision actually was, and how it might interact with one's own. Instead, perceived others were seen as hostile adversaries, immoral enemies, Blairites, or even Tories.

The goals of each side – political goals guided by an ethical vision – became subsumed within tactics that they calculated were necessary in order to gain control of the party. Focusing on the relationship between Ronny and Charles allowed me to add more detail on how such ethics played out not just within the politics of activist organizations but also within the ties between people. Moral critiques of state structures were affected by judgements of persons. And moral critiques of persons were affected by judgements of their roles in contesting, perpetuating or promoting particular ways of structuring state healthcare. Interpersonal relations, ethical reasoning and political contestation became inseparable. The battles between and within political organizations were waged by people. The various moral critiques intertwined and coalesced around the word, 'socialism'.

In Chapters 3 and 4, I explored how the NHS could be a focal point of solidarity, of a community uniting around a sense of shared interests that were institutionalized in a health service *for all*. But in this chapter, I have demonstrated the opposite. Actors' views on the structure of the NHS were used to inform judgements on whether a person was a good socialist. These evaluations fed into tactical decisions on whether or not to trust people and organizations. These evaluations were the basis on which coalitions formed or broke. In the SHA, I witnessed the latter.

The Labour Party, often described as a 'broad church', and itself formed from a coalition of various working-class societies (Hannah, 2018), saw cleavages open up within it between people who saw themselves as socialists and the other side as Blairites. Like Winant's (2019) description of the PMC in the Democratic Party, the moral antagonist that drew most suspicion and ire was neither the Tory, nor the capitalist, but the 'familiar enemy' *within* Labour itself. The suspicion that non-socialists or Blairites might undermine the goals of NHS activism – to advance towards a fairer society by countering cuts and privatization – handicapped the solidarity in numbers that the Labour Party was meant to enshrine. Familiar enemies battled each other for the Labour Party, rather than uniting to protect the public services they both valued more than the Tories did.

In December 2019, 15 months after I completed my fieldwork, the UK had another general election. The Tories won a landslide victory. The Labour Party won 202 seats, which represented a loss of 60 seats since the last election in 2017. It was Labour's worst election result since 1935. Corbyn announced his resignation the next day.

6

NHS Workers and Industrial Power: An Interview with Emma Runswick

In its first full year, the NHS employed 400,000 people, making it the country's third largest employer. By 1961 it was the largest, having overtaken the National Coal Board and the British Transport Commission (Saunders, 2016). Over the decades from 1948 until now, the number of staff has increased, spanning a bewildering array of clinical and non-clinical roles, and from a variety of educational, class, ethnic and national backgrounds. Despite the wide range of prestige, pay, security and influence among staff, the cultural resonance of the NHS has somehow allowed these disparate workers to identify with one another, as 'NHS workers' (Saunders, 2022). At times, NHS staff have mobilized this identity to their own ends, for example by linking industrial actions to efforts to defend the NHS.

Chapter 2 briefly touched on the issues faced by NHS workers during my fieldwork: inadequate staffing, high numbers of vacancies, low morale, burnout, bullying, excessive pressure, inadequate resources and moral injury. Further, one of the institutional responses to austerity was pay suppression. All of these issues contributed to a wave of strikes in 2022 and 2023, involving the British Dietetic Association, the British Dental Association (BDA), the British Medical Association (BMA), the Chartered Society of Physiotherapists (CSP), GMB (previously known as the General, Municipal, Boilermakers and Allied Trade Union), the Hospital Consultants and Specialists Association (HCSA), the Royal College of Midwives, the Royal College of Nursing (RCN), the Society of Radiographers, Unite and Unison.

Most in-house non-medical staff are employed on a contract framework known as Agenda for Change.[1] Most Agenda for Change staff received an improved pay offer following strikes, although many staff considered the offer still not good enough, since it did not restore their real terms pay to what it had been before austerity. Some rank-and-file organizations did emerge, such as NHS Workers Say No, to reject the improved pay offer. However, most union leaderships recommended acceptance of the deal. Member ballots in most unions did accept. Only the Royal College of Nursing and Unite rejected the deal. Since the majority of NHS staff were represented by unions that accepted, the offer was implemented in 2023.

The exception was the BMA, the doctors' union. Junior doctors and consultant doctors are employed on two separate contracts, completely separate from Agenda for Change. Consultants participated in strike action on four separate occasions in 2023 before accepting a new pay offer in 2024. Junior doctors participated in nine actions between 2023 and 2024, before accepting an offer from the new Labour government in July 2024. A new dispute was opened again in 2025, leading to three further strikes.

In this chapter, I present a lightly edited interview with Emma Runswick, junior doctor[2] and deputy chair of BMA Council. Emma and I discussed some of the arguments of this book as well as the industrial disputes that have taken place since my fieldwork. Previous chapters have touched on the problematic role of the BMA in relation to how it has interacted with the collective actions of other NHS workers.[3] In the interview, I also challenged Emma with these critiques of the BMA, both from the sociology of the professions, as well as from other campaigners.

I have chosen not to provide an analytic response to the interview for two reasons. First, out of respect for Emma, who was kind enough to lend me her time and give an on-the-record interview for this book. At times, Emma disagrees with me and some of the arguments of this book. I felt that me having the last word would be unfair. Second, our interview took place in April 2025, several years after my ethnographic fieldwork. Its place in this book is not as part of the ethnography. Rather, it provides a postscript, as well as an engagement with its findings from an interested actor: an NHS worker, an activist and a self-described socialist. As such, I take her words not as data for ethnographic analysis and incorporation into the argument, but as substrate for further reflection.

PP: Tell me who you are and what positions you hold.

ER: My name is Emma Runswick. I am a doctor training in psychiatry. I am in my fourth year of working in psychiatry. And I am also an elected official in the British Medical Association. I am deputy chair which is one of the four chief officer roles in the BMA.

PP: And can you tell me a bit more about yourself?

ER: I come from a trade union family background. My parents were active in the civil service unions and I grew up around that activity and the political activity associated with it. I identified as a trade unionist and socialist quite young and I started becoming active in the BMA in my first year of medical school. I have consistently organized with my colleagues locally. As I became active at a national level with people around the country, I have also worked for – what I would describe as – a more functional BMA in a trade union sense. A BMA that is capable of using leverage to win disputes and influence the policy and systems that that we work within, improve our own lives and therefore the lives of our patients and the communities that we serve. One of the things I have worked for has been basic democratic functioning in the union. Other activities have been more substantial. But I guess I am now most well known for the pay restoration campaign. That really started in 2018 at the back of the agreement of the last contract, but came to most people's attention in 2022.

In 2022 I was elected to be deputy chair of council.[4] I had been on council since 2018, having been elected as a student. When I was re-elected in 2022, the situation for the campaign was fairly critical in terms of the direction of the union and we had decided that one of us – when I say 'one of us' I mean one of the people in the Broad Left or Doctor's Vote[5] – needed to stand and I was the only person who met the criteria.

PP: What motivates you to be a doctor?

ER: Lots of things. So, I think it's probably worth splitting into what originally motivated me to be a doctor vs what now motivates me to be a doctor, because I think those are different. What originally motivated me to be a doctor was that I was interested in – and good at – science. I know it sounds silly but, in medicine, people are grateful for the things that you do. And so are you. You *also* feel fulfilled by the work that you do, because you are actually making improvements to something or to somebody. And you have long-term stability where you're always going to have a job. That was what drove me towards medicine.

Now it has become fairly apparent that the medicine that I imagined, of stable employment, high salary and constantly making improvements to people's lives doesn't really exist or certainly not in the way I imagined it. I tend to say that I love the work I do but I don't like the job. So if I separate out the things about the work that I love, it is fulfilling. People do mostly get better. I have skills that I use to improve and occasionally save people's lives. That's really great. It's challenging. We have a great team to work with, people from a whole variety of disciplines. We have really interesting patients who trust us and tell us their life stories. All of that is kind of fairly fundamental to medicine and I love that.

The things that I dislike are all about the job and they are not fundamental. They are not fixed. So the fact that in medicine we also have short, fixed term contracts, that there isn't stability, that there is no guarantee of the next stage of training, that you are forced to rotate through different places through different jobs, whether you like it or not, that you are often at the whims of your supervisors. Again, most of them are great, but some of them are terrible. You are again at the whims of whatever the current government is and the political choices that they make about your service and about your pay and conditions. And there are lots and lots of things here that I thought would be true about medicine, that drew me to medicine – like stability and long-term employment – that don't actually exist. But the things that I love about medicine are still pretty true.

And then I think there's something that is kind of specific to medicine here in the UK, which was a factor both then and now, which is that I think it's important to be able to do something that aligns with my values. I love the fact that I treat people for free. I love that. I think it's important to our society. I think if I hadn't done this, I would have looked for other public sector work. Because I don't really want to make money for somebody else.

Specifically I don't want to make money for somebody who already has money and wealth. I don't want to participate in the transfer of capital from a person with less to a person with more. The NHS is fairly foundational in my enjoyment of my work. It attracted me when I was a teenager and it still attracts me now.

PP: And what motivates you to do the work you do in the BMA?

ER: There are probably a couple of answers. I grew up around trade unionism and it has always been a part of my life. In some ways it was never a question that I was going to do trade union work, whatever job I did. And then there's a kind of second answer, which is about my politics. I'm a socialist. I believe that workers should have more control over their lives and that we have, you know, two primary classes in society. Even though I'm fairly well off within the working class, I'm part of the working class. And I believe that trade unions are one of the primary ways in which we even out the power imbalance between working people and people who own stuff: a working class and a ruling class. To a greater or lesser extent in every trade union but especially in the case of healthcare, that means advocating for the pay, terms, conditions, welfare and training of myself and my colleagues. As doctors and medical students it's also advocating for the care of the patients that we serve and the communities that we live in. The BMA has traditionally done that in a kind of very top-down lobbying way. Which I don't think is always the most effective. And I think that if we're going to do that effectively, we need to be a more effective trade union. All of those things go together. In that it's a service for me, it's a service for my colleagues, it's a wider political service.

PP: You just described yourself as working class. I think by that you mean someone who needs to work in order to survive. Is that right?

ER: Yes.

PP: In order to pay your rent or your mortgage, to buy your food, to do everything you need to do in order to actually survive, you have to work. You have the freedom to work. And the freedom to starve if you don't work.

ER: Yeah.

PP: In the class system that you described, there were two classes. Who's in the ruling class?

ER: The ruling class owns the ways in which society produces things or services. The traditional or easy way of understanding this is by looking at a product. Let's say you make thingamajigs. The person who owns the factory that makes the thingamajigs doesn't have to do any work, but makes money off selling the thingamajigs that other people have made by selling those things for more than he's paid the workers who made them. That person – who's not actually working but owns things and has wealth by owning things – creates more money for himself. By owning things. That person is in the ruling class. But in modern capitalism, it's far more complicated than the thingamajig that one business owner sells. There are entire systems of products, services, financial systems, where there isn't any money at all. The money is imaginary. Nevertheless, those people run the majority of society for their own benefit or for the benefit of a very small number of people, leaving the rest of us in various degrees of poor circumstances. Good examples of this might be financial commodities traders, people who own lots but again don't tend to have quote unquote 'cash money'. So, you know,

America's oligarchs, Bezos, Musk would be good examples. But there are many.

PP: One of the things that people often say about the BMA is that it's not a working-class union. It's a middle-class union. How do you respond to that?

ER: It is a union that represents some middle-class people. We represent an entire profession: student to retired and everybody in between, anybody who has medical qualifications. When I say there are two main classes, well, there's a significant chunk of BMA members who are petty bourgeois, i.e. who both work and own to some degree. So: partners in GP practices, people who are practising in the private sector as independent contractors sometimes own their own premises. Sometimes they are self-employed, although not always. There are definitely groups that we represent who are not working class, or not traditionally defined as working class.

That being said, particularly in general practice, they too suffer from the particular situation that we have in the UK where they cannot freely sell like most self-employed people can. They contract only to one group, which is the NHS. Therefore they have the same difficulties – or very similar difficulties – as many of us would have with an employer. They just have it through a slightly different contractual arrangement.

So I think it's perfectly reasonable for people to say this is a middle-class union. Yeah, some of us are. I don't think that changes the fundamental purpose of organizing in this way for the vast majority of us who are working in a situation where we don't own the means of our work. You know, even the best-off consultants are working. They're working people. Some of them might – through other means – have some ownership, but just because they're better off doesn't mean that they're ruling class.

PP: Why not?

ER: Because it's not about your relative income. Your class is about your relationship to the means of production, not whether you have a nice house. But the higher salary does mean that they might be able to have bought things that might mean that they could quite easily be people who do own things related to the means of production. For example, some doctors have become landlords, some people will open businesses. But many don't and won't and increasingly it would be difficult for them to do so unless they've got wealth from somewhere else already.

We have about 200,000 members in the BMA at the moment, in April 2025, and more than 70,000 of those are residents.

About 20,000 are medical students. Another several thousand are public health doctors, almost all of whom work in the public sector. Academics, SAS[6] doctors, there are a substantial number of us who are not in this better off position. But even when we are, we still don't own the hospital. We can't just open a practice by ourselves. You can't be a surgeon without a premises to operate in. And surgeons don't generally own their own premises and employ all the nurses, cleaners, operating department practitioners, and all of the other people who work there. They work in an environment that provides that.

PP: But the increased salary does mean that you could be in a position to actually go and do that.

ER: Sure. But the gap between the highest paid consultant and Bezos is far greater than the gap between the highest paid consultant and the homeless person on the street.

PP: I think one of the first times I met you, back in 2016, you and Steven Watkins referred to the BMA being more of a professional association than a union. What did you mean by that?

ER: Professional associations and trade unions both came to the UK at a similar kind of time, around 1830s, 1840s kind of time. We've got lots of unions growing out of the Chartist movement and the democratic movements. But we also have the professional associations, including the BMA in 1832. And all of these are designed for similar reasons. They're designed to collectively advocate for the people within them. That's the purpose of the trade unions and professional associations. But how they did so was very different. The BMA did not traditionally consider itself a user of industrial leverage. I mean the kinds of things that we would consider industrial action or big rallies or, you know, campaigns, public political activity. It has used the established power of doctors, on all sorts of issues. Some that are about patient safety, like the banning of chloroform in the very early days of the BMA and, much more recently, the banning of smoking in public places.

But to advocate for the pay, terms and conditions of doctors in hospitals or primary care settings is different. They had some degree of professional status. So they could lobby for that, they could negotiate that, they could argue for that without using the tools that a more traditional quote unquote 'working-class' profession might have to use.

Unfortunately, the doctors-in-the-back-rooms of political power strategy has not continued to work like that. I say unfortunately. That's up for argument, isn't it? Producing a beautiful policy report about how this is bad for patients and bad for doctors, or some combination of both, does not change things in the way that it might have changed things in the past. And therefore that kind of professional association work does not produce the results that that we need it to.

Sometimes it's very effective. For example, at the moment we are doing quite a lot of ethics work on the proposals around physician assisted dying and we've been very successful as a professional association, using our expertise and our position in society to advocate for protections for both patients and for doctors.

PP: Do you feel that that's changed now?

ER: Yes.

PP: How has that change come about?

ER: With deliberate and sincere and continuous effort and organizing by initially small groups of people. And then many thousands of people who knew that the BMA needed to change.

The BMA became a trade union in the 1970s after having been the host of the General Whitley Council, a kind of quote unquote 'neutral place' to have a negotiating group for all of the medical trade unions.[7] Many of the medical trade unions had either dissolved or merged in the years between the foundation of the NHS and the early 1970s. The BMA became a union alongside its professional association status. That was a change in name and in a whole variety of other ways but it continued mostly advocating on a professional association basis, even when we had strike action. So in 2015, 2016, when we had the junior doctors dispute that led to a ballot and strike action, the internal approach of the BMA was still very focused on lobbying.

When we have used trade union approaches it has felt foreign to the BMA. It has felt like they would rather be out of that situation as soon as possible. They see industrial action or any kind of dispute as an anomaly, a blip in the otherwise good relationships between them and employers or the state. The idea is that we can work together to solve problems with bosses rather than fundamentally having different interests and therefore being in struggle with them. More recently we are in the process of building on the foundation of the professional association, which works for the things that it works for and doesn't need to be messed with. The BMA can continue doing professional association things the way it has done for many years, for example, on physician assisted dying.

But we also need to create an organization that can use trade union tactics on a regular basis, where it's not scared of the use of collective tactics to achieve change. One of the phrases I used to hear a lot in the BMA is: Oh, you know, well, if we march members up that hill how will we get them down again? This is from senior elected officials, who are doctors, but also BMA staff. What they are referring to is an idea that if you engage in some kind of industrial activity as a union then we're going to need to go back to a position where everybody's calm and friendly again at the end, like nothing has happened, so we can get back to our quote unquote 'normal', which is that ongoing stakeholder relationship. And I hate that so much because it assumes that the status quo is good or desirable. And I don't think it is. We have a health system which is in real trouble. We have shoddy terms and conditions across the sector. Pay has been significantly cut. There are parts of the country where people still regularly crash their car on the way home from night shifts. The idea that getting back to that normal is what we want … I think we can get that idea in the bin. We should create an organization which is able to constantly use trade union tactics at a whole variety of different levels to improve the lives of ourselves, our colleagues and our patients.

PP: My fieldwork was back in 2017–2018. A lot has changed since then. We've been talking about turning the BMA into a fighting union and there have been multiple big fights. One of the developments was that there were junior strikes throughout 2023 and 2024. I think there were nine in total, culminating in an average 22% pay increase over two years. And there were also four consultant strikes in 2023. So can you give me a bit of an outline of how the strikes actually came about?

ER: The 22% figure is for England. There were also strikes in the devolved nations along with different solutions and different settlements. I think we had 55 days of strike action from doctors in in the UK.

How did it start? I guess out of the Vote No campaign in 2018. We had the contract dispute and strikes in 2015, 2016. That ended in the imposition of a contract, much improved from the one originally intended by Hunt,[8] but nevertheless an imposed contract in the October of 2016. And then over the next two years, the Junior Doctors Committee negotiated improvements to that contract on the back of the fact that we had rejected it and were, in some degree, perhaps laughably, but in some degree, working under protest. When the new version of the contract came back to members in a referendum in 2018, I was involved in a campaign for students to vote no. We thought it was completely inadequate on issues of safety, on issues of progression, particularly for those who are less than full-time for any reason, but that's mostly women, carers and disabled doctors.

One of the issues was that it locked us into a pay arrangement for four years which said we would get 2% a year, or at least 2% a year, and that could be revisited if there was a significant change in circumstances. Given the situation with Brexit, with a whole variety of other international and UK-specific economic factors, many of us could see that going really terribly for us and we tried to keep in touch with those people who had been on the no side of that argument. We wanted to maintain the ongoing organizing work, whether it was around that issue or a whole number of other issues that we had with the BMA as members, activists and reps. We obviously didn't predict that we would have a global pandemic that would kill hundreds of our colleagues and family members and that would cause humongous inflation that would completely wipe out the impact of the 2% pay award. And many of us as reps and local activists were very heavily involved in work to protect and appropriately compensate doctors who were working during COVID-19. Whether that was around arguments around masks and ventilation, whether it was about safe rotas, ensuring that we didn't spread COVID-19 through the hospital system, involving ourselves in discussions about isolation procedures and so on.

Also discussions about how to remunerate people who were on absolutely mad rotas that, amazingly, the national Junior Doctors Committee said were fine. They [the Junior Doctors Committee] agreed with the NHS that they would abandon most of our contractual safety provisions on hours, without any commitments on remuneration or compensation or promises for the future or anything. Just abandon us to the whims of our employers at local level, which I still haven't forgiven them for. And which made it very, very difficult. There's a really funny line actually in that agreement, that says NHS England or NHS Employers is grateful to the BMA and will consider this in future negotiations.

And then of course the following year they gave us another pay cut. That meant that in 2020 and 2021, those of us who were active – and indeed a whole wider profession – were angry. We were treated pretty atrociously. Careers disrupted, people redeployed from things they really needed to do, people held in jobs they really hated or couldn't hack. People shielded, people treated awfully when they had to shield. You know, removed from their jobs, sometimes unpaid, because they were shielding and there weren't appropriate protections for people who were health workers. And what do we do with those people separated from their families so they didn't infect their families for fear of killing them? When we had sod-all information about how we were going to rescue people from this terrible disease. And then, at the end of that, after all the claps and the banging on the pots and everything, there's another slap in the face, another pay cut, and there's still been no progress on many of the outstanding issues that were meant to be subject to working groups in the aftermath of the 2018 agreement.

So we were still organizing around terms and conditions issues, but also around pay, around political issues around public health. And in other unions there was a growing campaign, the Pay15 campaign, mostly for health workers. We wanted to join that campaign in the BMA. I say 'we'. I mean a group of people, mostly in the Broad Left but also other activists, wanted to join the Pay15 campaign that was growing in other unions. We advocated for that. We won that position at conference. And the BMA did nothing about it. The leadership of the BMA at that time thought that that was a ridiculous ask.

But at the same time we were developing the maths about how much we had lost against inflation. When we had had pay freezes or 1–2% pay increases, pay uplifts, what was that doing to our purchasing power against inflation? By the time we had finally achieved the position in the BMA that we would ask for 15%, it had become apparent that, really, our pay was down over 20% against inflation since 2008, since the beginning of austerity. We had lost about a fifth of our pay, slightly more than that. And we were not only having the fight within the BMA structures. We were also organizing a broader range of reps, producing communications for members, for our colleagues: like posters or memes or little videos of government ministers or from the conferences or, you know, newspaper headlines, that communicated to people that we had lost this amount of pay. We were so much worse off than the previous generation of doctors. That was impacting our staffing levels because people were (are) leaving to go to Australia or New Zealand where you can be paid better. And organizing around these ideas.

When the the BMA then finally puts out an official communication saying, 'We're asking for 15%', the response [from junior doctors], because we had been organizing, was no longer, 'Oh wow, 15%. That would be great.' It was: 'Why are you only asking for 15%?'

This organizing was primarily not me. I want to be super clear that this is not my work. Initially, you know, ten and then 20 and then 100 people put in the effort of changing people's understanding and shifting the idea about what might be acceptable and achievable. Eventually we got to the stage where we could say: 'Well, why can't we have pay restoration?' Medics4PayRestoration were advocating for changing the BMA. The Broad Left were publishing reports of meetings. It became accessible for people who had not understood the BMA before to understand the BMA. And DoctorsVote was formed. DoctorsVote was initially a small group of people, mostly anonymous, who had a collection of skills that enabled us to organize not just ten or 20 or 100 doctors around the idea of pay restoration, but many thousands of doctors around the idea of pay restoration, who were able to talk to their colleagues and to create a sea change in elections within the organization. That shifted the outcomes of the 2022 UK Council election and then subsequently the Junior Doctors Committee elections. That finally brought the BMA much more in line with the positions of members on the question of pay restoration.

So from the summer of 2022, organizing members and the BMA to be in a position to have a fight on pay was the priority. We got to that point in January or February 2023. We absolutely smashed the ballot thresholds created by the Trade Union Act 2016.[9] The highest turnout, the highest yes vote that had been seen in a national dispute. And then, of course, you have to take your action. You have to negotiate and you have to take your action. And in our case the negotiation didn't occur. The Conservative government basically declined to talk to us at all. Initially they declined to talk to us because: what was the point? We weren't going to go on strike. And then they said, 'Until you cancel your action, we're not going to talk to you.' They were in this Catch-22. Nevertheless, persistent, high turnout industrial action was completed safely, and produced the best public sector pay deal of that strike wave. We continued to take strike action for many months after other unions had settled, often for very poor settlements in my opinion. And we achieved something I think quite remarkable. Is it pay restoration? No.

Is it good enough? No. Is it pretty good compared to what we would have achieved previously and had achieved previously? Yes. Is it better than what many other unions and their members achieved in the same period? Also yes.

PP: With the pay campaigns, one of the things that was notable was the way in which the BMA consciously protected the interests of people who qualified in countries other than the UK. Often those doctors are not British themselves. Why was that important?

ER: We're an international workforce. About a quarter of doctors in any particular grade are international medical graduates.[10] If you don't include those people in the dispute, you lose. Quite fundamentally. You have to ensure that groups that are more vulnerable to pressure are protected. If you don't do that, then you have lost before you start. I am hyper-aware that I'm a ginger, white woman. To bring uncertain international colleagues with us, who might have a whole range of different experiences of trade unionism, what we required was other international colleagues to be reassuring in that space.

So people who had been involved in the 2016 dispute who were international colleagues wrote blogs, communicated with colleagues. People who had not been involved in that dispute but nevertheless had more security or better understanding of the legal position made serious efforts in their own groups, whether that's Facebook groups or WhatsApp groups or directly, colleague to colleague, talking about how strikes would achieve change. And also how we were going to make sure that strikes were safe, that they wouldn't be deported for taking strike action, that we would never take enough strike action for it to be difficult for them. We would never take more than ten days in a row because at ten days of unauthorized absence then it does become a problem.[11] We worked consistently and persistently on promoting the voices of international colleagues in official BMA communications videos. We ran webinars with immigration lawyers because they were part of the dispute and every part of every person who's part of the dispute is important. You need to make sure everybody is supported.

PP: You've clearly outlined that the way you win is by acting together and by including all of our colleagues, regardless of where they are from. And the practical steps taken by the BMA to manifest a sense that an injury to one is an injury to all. One of the noticeable aspects of the pay campaigns was that the BMA seemed to be suggesting that paying doctors more would be good for the NHS in general. At times the BMA seemed to be arguing that if the government gave us a large pay increase the government would be supporting the NHS, protecting the NHS, even saving the NHS. Do you remember where that aspect of the messaging came from?

ER: Yes. There are multiple different arguments to make for pay restoration or any improvement to doctors' or health workers' terms and conditions more generally. They face – and convince – different people. So, to doctors, we mostly talked about the generational unfairness of losing a significant amount of pay against inflation. It is fair to be paid what your colleagues were paid in 2008. Your job hasn't got any easier. You're not working less. If anything, you're working more. You can make that comparison and people are motivated by that feeling of a lack of fairness.

Most members of the public will not be motivated by that. And it is not the only argument. We have a particular position in the health service, which is that we are required to run it. Healthcare doesn't exist without doctors. We also have a situation where we are losing hundreds of doctors every year to abroad. For a whole variety of reasons but pay and conditions are significant in that. Mostly to Anglophone countries like Canada, Australia, New Zealand, Ireland, particularly Ireland from Northern Ireland. It is possible for all of these arguments to be true. It is unfair to pay doctors less. If you pay doctors less, they leave. That causes understaffing. That makes our jobs more difficult. But also it makes your healthcare worse. The healthcare that we can provide gets worse. It means we can do less. If we lose people who are more senior, we can't train people as easily. And that's a downward spiral.

If we retain health workers, not just doctors but all health workers, by treating them well, paying them appropriately, training them, having them in secure employment, then healthcare can improve. We can rebuild aspects of the health service that have largely collapsed through many years of underfunding, lack of resource, privatization, fragmentation and so on. So there are lots of things going on in this space. But the arguments that I and others who were representing the BMA to the public in news media focused on were those that would be useful for the majority of people who were consuming that media. And it was true. But it is also only one of the lines of argument that was used in this campaign.

PP: It sounds like you're saying that the argument around protecting the NHS was just about protecting the possibility of being able to provide health care at all rather than a symbolic idea of protecting the NHS or the specific way in which healthcare is structured here?

ER: Well, what happens when you have shortages? What has happened to the state of healthcare in this country over the last several years? As waiting lists increase, people who can pay to skip the queue do pay to skip the queue. That's what happens. So, you create an environment where you have a two-tier health system. So, if you want a system that provides free at the point of use healthcare on a timely basis, in order of need rather than ability to pay, you have to retain staff in your public health care system.

If you don't do that, then you will end up with a system which treats only the urgent and desperate in the public healthcare system. Those who want their elective care more quickly will get it privately. We've already moved quite a significant way along that line. It's not going to get any better if you lose all your doctors.

PP: It wasn't just an argument the BMA were using to convince the public. You do genuinely believe there is an intrinsic link between paying doctors enough, retaining them within the public health care system, and therefore being able to perpetuate the NHS.

ER: Yes, but what I'm saying is saving the NHS is not the *primary* argument that we're having when we're talking about pay restoration. And I think if you said that to most doctors in this campaign they would reject that being the primary purpose of the campaign. That was one of the primary communication experiences of doctors in 2015, 2016. Back then, the new contract was 'Not safe, not fair' and our action was about 'Saving the NHS'. But actually, most doctors don't like working in the NHS. The NHS is a crap employer. It treats us badly. We rotate frequently with no control over our lives. We have fixed term contracts. We uproot ourselves, often hundreds of miles across the country, to get a job, to progress. The pay is poor. It's almost never correct. We regularly get emergency taxed because the payroll systems are wrong. If we are less than full-time, we're unlikely to ever be paid correctly, even payslip to payslip, because it's consistently messed up. We have shoddy resources. Like, it's a regular joke, a meme, that junior doctors sit on bins because there are no functional chairs. We don't have appropriate IT systems or enough phones or enough staff to provide the care that we want.

The NHS is a bad employer. Right? Doctors are not out here being like, 'Oh, I love the NHS.' Most of us, right? Not me specifically, but most of us really hate working in the NHS. But that doesn't mean we don't have a kind of political commitment or a moral commitment to free at the point of use healthcare. It doesn't mean that it can't be part of advocating for improvements. But it is not the primary messaging for doctors.

PP: I just want to push back on that a bit because at the pickets and the protests, often there were chants and banners that put our employment within the NHS front and centre. There was something that appeared to be galvanizing about talking not just about being doctors and being underpaid, but that we were doctors *in the NHS*.

ER: Yes. But I don't think that conflicts. What I've just said is that doesn't get rid of the moral and political commitment to the NHS project.

PP: There was a pride as well. Pride to be NHS workers.

ER: Yes, 100%. You asked me at the beginning about why I am a doctor and I said there is something about being in a public service that provides healthcare for free, right? It 100% gives people pride. For sure, we talked about it and I talk about it and other doctors talk about it. Sometimes you hear me and others say a union that can win pay restoration can win anything. And when we say anything, we also mean a better system, a better service. But we're not out here defending the NHS as-it-is, because the NHS as-it-is is awful. We didn't throw all our eggs in that 'Save our NHS' basket because there are many people for whom, if the NHS was a different system, they wouldn't be unhappy. The NHS is not a good employer. So the arguments are diverse and they interlink and overlap. For sure, it is true that you have to retain doctors in the National Health Service in order to maintain the National Health Service for patients. But I think if what you've picked out of the pay campaign is 'Save the NHS', that's actually not what the pay campaign is for the vast majority of members of the BMA.

PP: But there is a moral and political commitment to the NHS.

ER: Yes.

PP: Not just for you but for members generally.

ER: And pride. You're right about the pride.

PP: So what is the relationship between that and the pay campaign?

ER: Well, I think I've described the link in terms of retention. There's a direct argument about retention and about recovery, particularly post pandemic. But I think there's also a more fundamental thing underneath, which is that if you care about the NHS, if you've got a moral or political commitment or a pride in working for the NHS, you do want it to work. Right? You want it to be good. We don't come to work to provide rubbish healthcare or, you know, not ring the family member, or hand over a massive list of jobs to your colleague that you haven't managed to get to today because you're understaffed. We all come to work to look after patients and we want to do it well. So there's something quite fundamental about taking control. And that's what happens in a strike. In a medical strike, we don't just leave patients to die. We decide who gets care. That's what happens in the strike. We decide what's emergency or critical or maternity care. You know, things that are going to happen now, right? All of those things keep happening. And the things that are less urgent get sidelined and that's a collective profession-wide decision about what's urgent and what's not urgent. What is okay to not do and what is not okay to not do. That's the shift that happens in a medical strike. It's not that people don't get care. It's that *who* gets care changes.

PP: Who does get care when we take strike action?

ER: The people who need it most. That's fundamentally what changes. And when you empower a whole group of people in that way, and clinical leaders and clinical teams have to take more control of the systems that they work in, they make improvements. So we have a reasonable amount of evidence now that during strike action bed flow is better. People are admitted and discharged more quickly. You know, quite remarkably, if you remove a section of people and suddenly all of the administration of the hospital is designed to facilitate what clinical leaders are saying is necessary – plus the fact that you've got more senior decision makers seeing patients earlier – healthcare improves. That sounds ridiculous but why does that happen? It happens because there is more clinical control.

When we have these arguments about how to structure healthcare or how to provide staff for healthcare or how to remunerate or how to treat people who work in healthcare, we are saying that it can be better than this. If we work together it can be better than this. So not only is it a direct and explicit link between 'If you pay us more there will be retention and then the NHS will have better services', underneath that there is 'If we collectively organize we can improve the service that we would all like to be proud of'.

So the BMA is committed to those moral principles of universal, free, comprehensive care. But it is resolutely not committed to the system working in exactly the same way that it currently works. It is committed to improving that system to better fit those moral principles and to make it a better place to work. And those things all fit together. Our working conditions are our patients' treatment conditions.

PP: So the NHS did play a role in the campaigns. What would you say to someone who accused doctors of weaponizing the NHS? Because it's free and well-loved and you work there, you and the BMA use that for your own benefit.

ER: Does that matter? If people want the health service then the tactics that people working in it use to improve the lot of their own lives and the services they provide … I'm not sure it matters what those tactics are. Just like London Underground workers weaponize that they run the entire capital. Well, yeah, that's their job. They drive the Tube or they run the stations and then they're on strike. You can't use it. That's the route that they've got.

PP: Why should a person who's not a doctor support our actions?

ER: If you are another worker of any kind, the successes of any group of workers is beneficial to you, any other group of workers. I support the Birmingham bin strike, not because I live in Birmingham or because I'm a refuse worker, but because if they win, it makes it more possible for other workers to win and for our entire class to improve their lives. If you are a person in the UK, then at some point in the past, present or future, you are going to be a user of healthcare. If you are going to be or are a user of healthcare, then you need health workers. We are some of those health workers. For us to provide you with good consistent care, we have got to have good conditions. So there's at least two arguments.

PP: The factors that led to wage suppression in the NHS actually affected many or most sectors. Now, following the strikes, in terms of purchasing power doctors' pay has returned closer to where it was than a lot of other workers. Your argument is that where we have had success, that will hopefully benefit workers' struggles in general, rather than just us. How can we make sure that those successes do spread? Is there a role for doctors to lead others into struggle for their benefit and possibly then our own mutual benefit. Do you see the BMA as potential leaders of a wider struggle?

ER: [Emma disputed the claim that doctors' purchasing power had improved more than other sectors of workers.]

Do I think that doctors should be leaders? I think we can be examples. But workers really have to lead themselves. Trade unionism is self-organization. I'm not going to wander into another union and tell them how to do their job, either clinically or how to organize themselves. Their situation will be specific to them. There is lots of crossover. Trade unionism has a science to it and an art to it. Lots of people have written about that, many of whom we have deliberately learned from, all around the globe. Things that are UK specific might be books like *Lessons in Organizing* (Little and Sharp, 2023) or *Workers Can Win* (Allinson, 2022). We can take things from what other people have done and learn from them for our own sectors and our own skills. We can and should interact with other trade unionists, but I think it would be counterproductive to say doctors are the leaders. Just in the same way that I think it's counterproductive to have a hierarchal, authoritative model in medicine, you know, where doctors are the 'leaders' who instruct patients, rather than experts collaborating with patients and other expert professionals.

PP: So any pay campaign, any campaign to improve terms and conditions for any group of workers, if successful will benefit other workers as well. And our working conditions are their treatment conditions. The implication being that advancing our own interests is likely to improve other workers' interests, and also is in line with improving patient conditions.

ER: Yes.

PP: I'm sure you'll agree that isn't always the case. There are times when those two things will be in conflict. So how do we negotiate that idea that, actually, as a union we are primarily advancing our own interests. If it's possible that our interests come into conflict with other workers' or patients' interests, how do we negotiate that conflict?

ER: In lots of different ways. In all groups of workers – doctors are no different – there are moral and political breaks for a whole variety of reasons. It might be in the interests of patients to reorganize services such that highly specialized services are all in one place, so that doctors can do a high enough volume of those cases to keep up their skills. But doctors might not want to move to the new place or lose access to the procedure that they occasionally do.

Normally, that splits opinion among the doctors. Hardly ever do we have a situation where there is a hard split between doctors and patients. In that situation, there will be a group of patients who are campaigning for their services to stay where they are because they're nearby. There will be a group of doctors who want to continue providing that service in that place because that's where they live and work. There will be a group of patients who say yes, we should run our highly specialist service in a central location and it's okay that we need to be in the ambulance for like five minutes longer. And a group of doctors who say yes, this is the very sensible thing to do to maintain our clinical expertise and I'm okay with not doing that anymore because it's something that I don't do enough to maintain my clinical expertise. So it stops being a unified position and starts being a complex negotiation of all of those factors.

There are some things where there's a more profession-wide approach on a patient safety issue. An example of that might be the associate professionals. Having failed as a profession, for a whole number of reasons, to put in place a scope of practice that was appropriate for associate professionals' level of training, we now have a movement against their existence as a profession.[12] That is a severe conflict with another group of workers. But in that case doctors are aligning themselves with patients' interests even when that can be quite personally difficult. Doctors who have taken on physician associates or anaesthetic associates in their department have looked at the outcomes, where the confusion around what their job is or what the training is has been put in Coroner Regulation 28 reports.[13] Resident doctors are saying, 'This person's often making mistakes and doesn't understand the limits of their knowledge. They come and ask me to prescribe something and then when I go and see the patient that's clearly not the right course of action'. Doctors are responding by limiting the scope of those people and/or no longer having them in their departments or by engaging with their professional bodies, for example, the Royal Colleges, to further limit the scope of practice of associate professionals. Through no fault of their own these professionals do not have the training to do the tasks that they have been given. That is creating a scenario where associate professionals are losing their jobs or are losing the extent of the jobs that they had previously. Here, doctors are putting themselves on the side of patients. Patients deserve good health care that is not being provided under this system with associates and therefore we are going to limit the ability of these people to do harm or to not do enough good. But the other side of the argument is: doctors would be better placed. Those are two very different examples where there might be conflict. In both cases we've got splits in the profession and different alignments of interests that intersect or conflict or align, and we negotiate those as a profession among ourselves and with the other parties in play.

PP: Those are great examples. The other one that I was thinking of was pay beds in the NHS, where there were strikes by nurses in the 1960s or 1970s against the existence of pay beds in the NHS, but doctors resisted those strikes. They didn't support those nurses because it was in doctors' interests to have these beds in the NHS that doctors got extra pay from. So that was part of the standard NHS consultant contract. But with marketization now, private contractors that are providing NHS services are often able to pay consultants pretty high salaries, but the other employees within those organizations aren't on such attractive conditions.

ER: Increasingly in the BMA we're seeing many local disputes about outsourcing. Hospitals' accounting offices will often be able to pay an outsourcing company more than they would pay for a wait list initiative[14] with their internal staff. For example, the surgeons, anaesthetists, cleaners and people who work in the hospital every day will not be paid sufficiently to motivate them to take up a Saturday list. But they will pay lots for external people to come in under the outsourcing company and use the theatre on a Saturday. And if there are any complications from that, all of the usual workers have to deal with those complications, while the outsourced visiting surgeon then sods off again. All of the benefits have been privatized and the losses are for everybody else.

We are now seeing several disputes about basically exactly that. There is a dispute in London where consultant anaesthetists stopped taking any additional work. The main point of their claim was about the use of external staff and outsourced companies. They wanted that to end and for the NHS to preferentially use internal groups of all staff. Because it's safer for patients; it reduces the complication rate when you use internal staff. People don't come into their theatre to find everything's been moved and messed up because some random person has rearranged things.

We are better training reps and empowering doctors to have fights not just about pay issues, but about wider issues like equality and bullying and the structure of services. You know, the things that doctors care about are much wider than pay. It's often about patient care, about the structure of services, about efficiency. Collectively, people can begin to challenge what's happening in their area.

PP: So some of these debates about the alignment of interests are missing the point that the way in which we consider or conceive of what our interests are in the first place isn't set in stone. It's not an objective thing. It is subjectively defined and some of it depends on who we consider the group who we consider 'us' to be.

ER: Yes. And it is definitely true that there is a within-profession split. Or between-professions split. Those are not always concrete lines.

PP: So some of the work is on how we define what our interests are and also how we work on particular alliances to broaden our sense of what our interests *could* be.

ER: Yes and also what we collectively decide our positions are as an organization. In the BMA we want an NHS as we previously described it: publicly run, publicly accountable, free at the point of use, high quality. Therefore, where there are splits in interests, as a union we have something collectively agreed to fall back on. We're going to back the things that are politically aligned. So, you know, in the discussion about: are we going to back the doctors who are making absolutely loads of money from an outsourced company or are we going to back the doctors who are saying this is far less safe than if you used internal staff for less money, it's an accounting function. You would probably spend less money and have fewer complications and it would be better for patients and staff if you insourced work rather than outsourced work. Well, we're going to back that group.

If we've got a disagreement about how to restructure services, like highly specialized services being centralized, then we're probably going to negotiate some kind of compromise agreement. We've got to be part of negotiations for those who want to move and those that don't, getting the best outcome for as many individuals as we can from that change.

The overall aim is that our services get better. But we don't accept that services only get better if we deteriorate our pay and conditions. We sometimes hear arguments from the government, like, 'You're striking against patients'. Or, 'If we pay you, it's a zero-sum game that has to come from patients or from services', which is just a lie. It's political choices that are making those decisions. We don't have to accept that. Where there are conflicts we have to diligently work through them. But I don't accept that there is a fundamental conflict between the interests of doctors and of other health workers or between doctors and patients.

PP: I think that's a good point to move on to alliances and coalitions. Tell me about your and the BMA's work with other unions and why that's important.

ER: The BMA is not in any kind of trade union organization, like the Trades Union Congress. Nor are we Labour Party affiliated. But we have tried to work with other unions increasingly over the last couple of years. Previous to this leadership, we've held ourselves out to be very independent, perhaps not even part of the labour movement. I see the BMA as part of the UK labour movement. I want us to be involved in that. There are some things which we have done for a long time, like NHS Staff Council where we and other NHS unions interact together with employers over things that are shared, but mostly over things related to Agenda for Change. So there is some teamwork there on, for example, the NHS Handbook, which has maternity provisions and things in it. But there is also a lot of letting the Agenda for Change unions do their own thing. The separation of our contracts and our pay structures means that the work isn't as close as the other unions are to each other. It also means there's far less conflict because we don't have different positions about what their contract should be.

At any given point it allows us to work as closely as we can with any or all of the other health unions. That has meant that we have coordinated industrial action with, for example, the Society of Radiographers. We have worked quite closely with the Royal College of Nursing. It was really the timing of their dispute, and their capitulation on demands, that separated us rather than us not wanting to work with them. We have talked to many unions around upcoming campaigns, not just on pay but on wider issues like trade union legislation.

So we have okay relationships with the other unions. At local level, we now have pan-union disputes. So that shift from occasional national BMA industrial action to empowering local activists and reps to do things has meant that there is now an all-health-union dispute in South Tees about the introduction of a parking fine system. All workers who work at that trust are involved in that dispute, not just the BMA. Because it's a pan-union discussion, it isn't going to be solved by, you know, privileges for consultants. That's not going to be the solution to this set of problems because we are working together at local level much better than we have done previously. So our relationships are, I think, fair. There's also the British Dental Association, the dentists, who we work with hand and glove. We've got a much closer relationship with them because we share some services.

But there's also probably something to say about the fact that we're now quite politically different. BMA officers are all working doctors whereas in other healthcare unions they are mostly professionalized trade union officials, no longer doing clinical work. That creates a gap between our union and other unions. The fact that we are driving forward quite a radical program creates a gap between us and most of the other unions. Our belief is that coordination and collaboration between the unions makes us all stronger. But we're not prepared to absolutely hobble our own strategy in order to make that work. We're going to progress our aims as the BMA. If we can work with others on that programme, great. If they're not there and they're, you know, going to continually fold at early stages of conflicts then that's on them.

PP: You mentioned that the BMA is not a member of the TUC. Tell me more about that.

ER: I've been an advocate for us to join the TUC for a long time. But it has now been lost at the national conference twice. I mean a motion has been submitted suggesting joining the TUC, and the vote has not gone in favour. Both in 2016 and then more recently, I think in 2023. In 2016 it was mostly: 'Oh gosh, we can't possibly join those left-wing radicals.' In 2023 the argument had completely flipped to: 'Well, we're being very effective without being in the TUC. Most of those TUC unions have folded or sold out.' And: 'It's a lot of money. Why would we bother?'

I think there's a fair amount of truth in the idea that the TUC has not been as effective or useful as it as it could have been in the in the last couple of decades, under the Labour government and then coalition and Tory austerity. I don't think workers of any kind are required to do things that are not useful for them. So I understand the arguments. That being said, I would prefer much greater collaboration across the labour movement. I think it's outrageous that some unions have been able to sue and punish other unions for recruiting in their own sectors, for example. I think it's ridiculous how unions compete with one another. I think we'd be in a much better place as a class and as a labour movement if we had more collaboration.

PP: I'm going to move on to the critiques of the BMA from various quarters. I'll start with the right-wing critique. The right-wing critique is that the BMA is actually very powerful. Doctors are already highly paid and any campaigns for even higher pay are just evidence of greed. And also that the BMA gets in the way of meaningful reform of the NHS.

ER: Okay. With what evidence? Like the BMA is so powerful that our wages were cut by almost a third. The BMA is so powerful that the NHS has been crumbling around us for about a decade, both metaphorically in terms of services and also literally, in terms of our buildings falling down with RAAC[15] and asbestos, crumbling buildings that were built in the … whenever they were built. And the BMA is so powerful that we've got more than seven million people on waiting lists.

It's clearly nonsense, right? Clearly nonsense. Have we had some influence on some things? Yes. Have we had some successes in making things not as bad as they could have been? Yes. Have we improved some things for ourselves and for patients? Sure. But what I was talking about before in the professional association side is that although it's useful for some things – smoking and assisted dying being two recent examples – fundamentally, we haven't been powerful enough. Now we are organizing in a way which makes us more powerful and I hope it continues to make us more powerful because we can be advocates not just for ourselves but also for the patients and services that we run.

PP: The left-wing critique is that despite consciously indexing our interests with those of the NHS and other NHS workers more broadly, the BMA and doctors' interests are not the same as other NHS workers, nor workers in general. And the BMA gets what it wants, gets an increased pay offer, and then withdraws, rather than acting in mutual solidarity with other workers.

ER: Okay, that's also not based in reality. What happened in the recent disputes? Who withdrew from disputes? It wasn't us, it was other NHS workers, including when we were trying to work with them. The Agenda for Change unions mostly took 5%. They withdrew from the disputes well before we did, and we would have continued to support them in their disputes, including with collaborative coordinated action, had they stayed in dispute. That they chose to withdraw is not on us. The fact that when we then won more, other unions criticized us, is quite outrageous. We had quite a lot of comment from the Royal College of Nursing about, 'How dare the government pay doctors so much when they only gave nurses 5%.' Well, the RCN recommended 5%. And the RCN's members voted for it or in many cases didn't vote for it, but that's what you negotiated and what you were prepared to win, prepared to strategize to win.

We weren't prepared to settle at 5% and we fought for more and we won. And we would have been alongside the RCN if they were still in the fight. The idea that doctors' interests are fundamentally different to other workers' interests is also just false. Like, in what way do nurses not care about better terms and conditions, better staffing, better pay, better patient care, care by the right people? High quality buildings, quick, timely care. Do nurses not care about that? Doctors care about those things. I think nurses care about those things as well. And more than that, I think almost all workers will care about that, as users of the health service. But also they will have equivalent things in their own industries and sectors that they care about.

PP: So the BMA will act in solidarity with other unions, other workers, but primarily the struggle has to come from the workers themselves?

ER: Yes. The BMA can't do that fighting for them. Although the BMA will stand with them 100%. And indeed, some of us are really trying to assist people in other unions to do that, through networks like Troublemakers at Work. Or through political organizations or through campaigning organizations, individual activists and doctors are supporting NHS Workers Say No and other organizations to improve mutual organization. So, it's about sharing skills, sharing organization, particularly at grassroots level.

PP: The academic critique from the sociology of the professions is that health politics is conventionally seen as tripartite. We have the population, the state and then organized medical interests, whether that's the professional associations, the Royal Colleges, the BMA, etc. Putting it that way clearly outlines how doctors' interests aren't always the same as those of patients or the public because they might have differing views on how those things are organized. Given doctors' class position, is that indexing of medical interests with the public, for example through the use of arguments about saving the NHS, is it not a smoke screen for advancing doctors' own interests at the expense of those with less power or influence or leverage?

ER: I'm not sure I would accept that they are separate. In the negotiations around organization of healthcare or pay or conditions or whatever, actually there are only two groups in the room and the public isn't one of them. It's the state or NHS Employers or the Department of Health and the organized groups of health workers of whatever kind. In that discussion, both sides of the negotiation claim to be on the side of patients. I think most people would accept that doctors care far more about patients and patient care than politicians do, in the vast majority of cases. We are closer to the care that we provide.

As I said, all of our elected officials are still working as doctors. We know what the impact is of their political decisions. Often serious harm, right? Serious harm comes from their decisions and we have sight of that and knowledge of that. So although both sides will claim to be advocating for patients, and sometimes maybe they genuinely believe that they are, I truly think that in that discussion it is doctors who are aligned with patient interests. Even if that doesn't necessarily mean that it costs less, from the taxpayer perspective.

In that space, in discussions between patients, the public and government, doctors are in the working class. We discussed the exceptions to that but we weren't kidding when we said that junior doctors, Foundation Year 1[16] doctors at the beginning of this dispute were paid less than £15 an hour. The minimum wage from this April is 25K[17] a year for somebody full-time. Medical wages are not that much higher than that, particularly in the lowest grades. It is absolutely ridiculous to suggest that those people are somehow separate from other workers. You know, not an absolute minimum wage, but not that far from it to be honest. I don't think it's correct to suggest even that the best paid consultants are fundamentally separate. Are many of our members part of a better off layer of the working class? Yes. But I don't think their interests are fundamentally different.

I challenged the premise of the tripartite model but then I haven't answered the question! Is it a smoke screen for advancing our interests at the expense of those with less power, influence, or leverage? No. Doctors regularly advocate on behalf of people with substantially less power and influence. As individuals, but also as a group. This is a professional association side example: right now the BMA is being very influential in the discussion about physician assisted dying. We are firmly on the side of good palliative care, measures against coercion, no requirement to bring it up in the way that they do in some places, like Canada. But equally no prohibition, so that people have equitable access to the service.

In the BMA we have a patient liaison group which sends a representative to every committee meeting. We deliberately and consistently integrate patient needs into our own advocacy because that is what's important to doctors. It's part of the professional ethos.

I was talking about what do I like about the job? Well, what do I like about medicine? What do I value about the work that I do? Patients are a blooming big part of it. And that's basically all of us. All of us have that approach. Almost all. There are people who are burnt out who no longer have that approach but basically all of us started with a we-can-help-people perspective. I don't think that goes away.

PP: If you combine the academic and the left-wing critiques, you get one that's close to one of the core anxieties that activists in my fieldwork were actually worried about. They were worried that they were increasingly defending something indefensible because they were they were trying to defend the NHS or some idea of the NHS. For them that didn't mean just keeping it the way it is. It was about improving the NHS. But sometimes it did literally mean resisting a change to the NHS. Say, a cut or a new model of care that they felt actually wasn't going to be beneficial. So, it was literally keeping the NHS as it was, while at the same time recognizing that the NHS is not good enough as it is. So, one activist referred to that as defending the indefensible. We're increasingly being put in a position of defending the indefensible.

They were mostly referring to cuts making the services provided by the NHS worse. Being put in a position of defending a structure that actually provided worse outcomes than it used to. And the book also explores how the NHS kitemark has become a source of stable revenue for private capital. Outsourced NHS services are provided by a private company that is often owned by private equity. Capitalists have invested quite heavily in providers of NHS care over the last decade or so, especially in psychiatry, where we've got entire hospitals of NHS patients in the private sector. So if activists are campaigning for more NHS funding, then they're actually simultaneously campaigning for more funds being siphoned into the private sector.

That wasn't something that they voiced at the time of my fieldwork, but it is something that is happening more and more in the political economy of the NHS. The more state funding is dedicated to the NHS now, the more wealth is redistributed upwards via the private sector.

And then finally, we have the example of the BMA putting the defence of the NHS front and centre of its arguments, to increase doctors' pay, when doctors – and specifically consultants – are already among the highest paid workers in the NHS. So that indexing of doctors' interests with those of the NHS possibly serves to harness the public image of the NHS as an example of socialism, equality, justice while actually using it to consolidate the already superior income of its highest paid professionals. Is the BMA taking active steps to recognize that danger. Is it a danger?

ER: I don't think that consultants being highly paid is a danger to the NHS as a project. They're highly paid for good reason. Even if you didn't think that the level of responsibility and training that they have entitles them to be well paid, if you don't pay them, they move. So, you kind of have to. We exist in a world where you can get paid double what we pay in the NHS if you go and work in Australia. And that is absolutely decimating the national health service in Northern Ireland. Because you could work half the time over the border and get paid the same.

Do I think higher pay for consultants is a threat? No. Do I think that advocating for more funding for the NHS is inherently advocating for upwards wealth redistribution via the private sector? No, I don't. I think you can make both arguments. We are capable of walking and chewing gum at the same time.

We can advocate for a publicly accountable, publicly provided, well funded, well resourced, well staffed NHS. And we should do. And the vast majority of people in this space are doing so, whether they are in organized unions in the BMA, outside the BMA, in campaign groups, I don't think anybody is not asking for it to be publicly provided. We are aware that money is being diverted in this way in the NHS. In the BMA we call that waste. Money is being wasted. Because if it's pocketed into profits, it's not being used on patient care and that's wasteful, right? Most patient care is staff wages. That's okay. People deserve pay for the work they do. But it is wasteful to put public money in the pockets of people who are doing no work for the NHS, instead of people who work for the NHS.

I don't just mean clinicians. I also mean people who ring up and book appointments, people who run the IT, people who clean, people who port people from place to place. You know, all of the variety of people who do estates maintenance or whatever. All of those people are part of the public system. We could have more of them and better conditions, and therefore better maintenance and improvement of our services if we spent money in the service rather than diverting it into the private sector.

The BMA is hyper-aware of that and we say it regularly. And increasingly we are creating the power at a local level to challenge where that happens, because lots of the decisions that are being made about outsourcing or privatization are made at a local or regional level and therefore that's where they need to be challenged. We are beginning to get the ability to do that in a way that we haven't had before.

So even when we came out against the Health and Social Care Act in 2012, what did we actually do? What did the BMA do in that period? We said it was bad. We maybe sent some people to demonstrations. Did we prevent any of it from happening? No. Because we didn't have that power. The professional association was not sufficient to stop the political power of government from fundamentally destabilizing our health service. What would be powerful enough is collective action by the most senior, well-paid groups of workers in the NHS to prevent or reverse decisions that cause privatization or outsourcing decisions. That would be powerful enough. We have the opportunity to develop that power as a more effective, more functional trade union, not just a professional association.

PP: You said if you weren't a doctor, you'd be some sort of other public sector worker. You support public services. Most other public services don't have the adulation that the NHS has. Why is that? Is the NHS more important than other state institutions? One of the arguments of the book is that it's important partly because it's one of the aspects of the socialist welfare state that actually is still standing. And that part of that symbolic importance is also around the fact that the reason it's still standing is because people have fought for it.

ER: I think there are lots of parts of the state that still exist and that people have fought for. And there are lots of examples of things that have been lost like British Telecom, Royal Mail, you know, things that are no longer ours collectively. There's something about the NHS which is ours. I'm not really sure exactly what that is, but it's something about it being a shared resource for all of us. Yeah. Not certain. I'm very happy to say this though. It's definitely one of the most significant aspects of socialist infrastructure. It's one of the biggest employers in the world. It treats millions of people every year. It has prevented millions of deaths through vaccination programmes and prevention.

It saves lives on a regular basis, as well as improving them. Everybody interacts with it. It's a demonstration of a socialist idea of collectivism and collective ownership without it being a kind of insurance. People pay in what they can and they take out what they need.

That's something quite special. Its universality separates it from most other aspects of the state. With the special nature of illness and becoming unwell, the element of it being collectivized and shared and owned by all of us ... that generates the fact that people are prepared to fight for it and are so vitally and fundamentally opposed to privatization.

It feels like a moral terror to profit from people's illness. You know, from the very beginning Bevan said it'll last as long as there are folk with the faith left to fight for it, right?[18] Those things are all running through the cultural importance, the status that it achieves by being part of the socialist welfare state: the fact that people fight for it, the fact that it has survived several rounds of very right wing government when other major British institutions have not done, the fact that it's universal in a way that lots of other services are not. All of those things come together to make it a site of very serious ongoing struggle to improve the bits of it that still stand and to regain the bits that we've lost. It's crucial.

Conclusion

> Stay at home. Protect the NHS. Save lives.
>
> *UK government communication during COVID-19 lockdown, April 2020*

I wrote the conclusion of the doctoral thesis on which this book is based in the summer of 2020, while the world was still in the thick of the pandemic. At the time, the preceding chapters read as the unfolding of a tragedy. In December 2019, Labour suffered a landslide election defeat. In January 2020, parliament passed the European Union (Withdrawal Agreement) Act. In the same month, the UK had its first confirmed cases of COVID-19. The first confirmed death as a result of COVID-19 occurred in early March. By 30 June there had been 50,574 deaths as a result of COVID-19 (Office for National Statistics, 2020). The inadequacies of the state's pandemic response – rooted in austerity, fragmentation and privatization – were painfully exposed. As summarized by the Institute for Public Policy Research, 'the UK system was in a poor position to resist a health shock … The fact that the UK's health and care system has struggled during the coronavirus pandemic can be traced back to decisions taken during austerity … COVID-19 has shown the consequences of these cuts' (Thomas, 2020: 3).

The government implored us to 'Stay home. Protect the NHS. Save lives.' I saw these three short sentences on billboards, on TV, in email signatures, on websites. Prime Minister Boris Johnson sent a letter to all UK households with the same message. What were Boris Johnson and Matt Hancock talking about when they talked about the NHS? What could it mean that they, just like the activists with whom I had spent so much time thinking, observing and campaigning, referred to *protecting* the NHS?

The central claim of this book has been that the NHS operates as a moral example that draws its strength not just from its role as a symbol, but also from the fact of its ongoing existence as an actually existing state structure, remembered and imagined in particular ways by particular people with particular effects on the creation or cleavage of ties between social groups. My argument is a useful vantage point from which to survey the pandemic's intensification of discussions regarding the NHS, the state, the state's obligations and what it means to show solidarity with one's fellow citizens. Most importantly, Johnson and Hancock's rhetoric provides further evidence that the *meaning* of the NHS was precisely the focus of this ethnography's ethicopolitical conflict – what I, following Ginsburg (1989), have called interpretive battles. In this concluding chapter, I summarize the arguments of the preceding chapters, and relate them back to the moral economy framework that has been whirring away in the background.

The moral economy of NHS activism

In the opening pages of this book, I posed the question of what the NHS *is*. I wondered how an answer to this question might relate to other questions, such as what activists imagine it to be, what it was, what it could be or what it ought to be. In the Chapter 1, I answered the question of what it is in a way that set up further questions on social relations that were answered in subsequent chapters. How does the moral imagination of the NHS become the focus of an interpretive battle? How do sides form in the battle? What kind of social relations emerge in these battles, what coalitions, what cleavages?

Activists understood the history of the NHS, of neoliberalism, of cuts and privatization within the contexts of their own life histories. Many of them were in their 50s or 60s; they considered themselves 'children of the NHS'. They remembered how they had benefited from state welfare, growing up in a society in which state services were one illustration of how members of society took responsibility for one another. They drew on these memories to imagine the NHS as a moral example of 'actually existing socialism', by which they meant a realization of socialist values, 'the social fabric', as Leroy described socialism. The NHS demonstrated not only how the state ought to intervene to foster a society in which citizens took responsibility for one another, but also demonstrated that the state *could* intervene in such a way. Unlike the moral examples studied by Joel Robbins (2015), which are enacted in ritual spaces, the NHS's moral force derived from its embeddedness in everyday political and clinical life. This grip on the imagination made reforms a site of intense moral scrutiny: any change to its structure threatened an example of what the good society might look like.

They mobilized this understanding of the NHS – icon *and* existing structure – to interpret and contest the changes they were witnessing in the present. In so doing, they drew themselves into the evolving history of the interpretive battles over the meaning of the NHS. In Chapter 3, I interpreted activists' fears of privatization as a critique of the vulnerability of the state in the face of global capital. Activists understood that the hands of state actors were tied; even if managers and politicians stated that they did not want to privatize services, they would eventually be forced. Therefore, activists did not only look for and find possible pathways to privatization that might be opened up by reforms. They also predicted that those pathways would be followed. Market logics would prevail.

However, their critique was hampered by their mode of analysis. They had good reason to see danger in reforms that would tamper with the existing structure of the NHS. But the drive to protect the institution that they understood as the template for a good society diverted their attention from the vulnerability in the existing structure itself. When capital came for general practice, activists were blindsided.

Their memories of past privatizations went beyond mere confirmation of their fears. Activists also harboured 'collective memories of struggle' (Schmidt, 2015: 30) that added another layer to the symbolism of the NHS. They remembered resisting past attempts at privatization, with at least partial success, and understood this resistance as one of the reasons that the NHS still existed. The state was vulnerable, but the NHS, as activists imagined it, stood out from other public services precisely because it represented the capacity of the state to stand up to the power of private capital in the name of the public good, *as long as* it was supported by activists. As the Socialist Party pamphlet that Leon gave me said, 'If we fight, we can win.' Despite all this, activists were also aware that the first part of the sentence was a genuine protasis, that is, the 'If' was a genuine if. Activists feared that the direction of travel was towards catastrophe, increasingly difficult to resist, as private companies had consolidated their position in de-risked contracts providing state services including healthcare. As Galen put it, they were being pushed to defend the indefensible.

Who was the 'we' in the Socialist Party pamphlet quotation? How did it constitute itself, against whom? In his description of the moral economy of eighteenth-century food riots, Thompson (1991a) described how peasants and workers of different backgrounds developed an understanding that their interests were the same as one another; they formed a community of interests. In the moral economy of twenty-first-century healthcare activism, the universality of the NHS was central to the ethical system that underpinned Dunning KONP and Greater Manchester KONP members' arguments. The health service was universal insofar as it ought to provide care for everyone. Activists contested contemporary reforms that undermined their expansive understanding of the value – and practice – of universality in the NHS, such as the introduction of charges for 'overseas visitors'.

The activists that I knew thus considered themselves to be in alliance with the whole population of the UK. Anyone working to undermine such a conceptualization of the NHS was an opponent. Chapter 4 explored the puzzle of how it could be possible for activists, managers and politicians to express the same values in relation to the NHS, and yet be in battle with one another. Each side was frustrated by the other. Activists felt evaded and silenced by the managers and politicians. Managers and politicians evaded and silenced activists because they felt campaigners were hindering their genuine attempts to save the NHS. But just as Matt Hancock and Boris Johnson were not talking about the same thing when they referred to protecting the NHS, each side were talking about protecting different things in the political battles in Dunning and Manchester.

In the temporalities of managers and politicians, their scope to make comparisons to the past or to make long term predictions for the future was limited by their responsibility to make sure some kind of service continued in the immediate future. The difficulties of fulfilling this responsibility had been acutely sharpened by austerity. Therefore managers focused on reducing demand – and thus expenditure – to save the NHS. When they spoke of saving the NHS, what they were talking about was different from what activists were talking about. Their conception of the NHS only extended as far as they imagined was possible within the financial envelope that national government provided.

Activists contested the ideological closure inherent in such an imagination of the NHS. For them, the actual or predicted reduction in hospital capacity represented a failure of the state to meet a previously held obligation. This perceived abdication of an obligation acted as a metonym for cuts and privatization in all public services since 2010, when the Tory and Liberal Democrat coalition came to power. Failing on this obligation was a demonstration to activists that the government was remaking society in a way that they morally disapproved of. Insofar as the NHS was an example of how the state could and should intervene in society to facilitate its members taking responsibility for one another, cuts to the NHS represented a relinquishment by the society of that responsibility.

These shifts in the ways that people understood the state and its obligations were the basis for bringing forth new social relations. For Thompson (1991a), the process of protesting the price of bread contributed to the development of a class consensus in eighteenth-century England that state structures and laws – as well as the class that controlled such structures – were immoral. That consensus was uneven and inconsistent, yet forceful enough to bubble up into riots at times.

In Greater Manchester's NHS activism, protesting cuts and privatization contributed to a sense that NHS managers and local politicians were not on the same side of the moral argument as activists and the public. The moral antagonists here were the upper echelons of NHS England management in London, and the Tory Party politicians who were making decisions to reduce budgets. However, NHS activists felt that Dunning's councillors and managers were implicitly allying themselves with the decision-makers in London by failing to challenge the limits set by them.

Attributions of responsibility for reforms contributed to the formation of sides in a political battle. But such attributions intertwined with individualized evaluations of persons such that potential alliances sometimes turned to cleavages as people and/or organizations were perceived to betray other people, organizations and their ethical visions of the NHS. Chapter 5 explored and historicized such (mis)attributions within the Labour Party. While I never confirmed if people's suspicions of foul play or betrayal were well-placed, it was clear that mistrust was self-perpetuating. These moralized evaluations fractured coalitions that might otherwise have defended public services more effectively.

The suspicion that non-socialists or Blairites might undermine the goals of NHS activism – to advance towards a fairer society by countering cuts and privatization – handicapped the solidarity in numbers that the Labour Party was meant to enshrine. Familiar enemies battled each other for the Labour Party, rather than uniting to protect the public services they both valued more than the Tories did. Opportunities to build solidaristic coalitions were squandered.

In the final chapter, Emma Runswick, deputy chair of the British Medical Association Council, challenged some of my anxieties. She argued that doctors' battles for pay could coexist with a struggle for a publicly provided service and emphasized that high consultant salaries are not the threat; outsourcing and profiteering are. Her perspective underscored that class politics and trade unionism remain vital avenues for resisting privatization and that ethical visions of solidarity can inform union strategy.

Moral anthropology, moral economy and class

In the Introduction, I highlighted how moral anthropology has been criticized for making little space for political conflict (Kapferer and Gold, 2018; Narotzky, 2019), and for side-stepping issues relating to power and inequality (Ortner, 2016). I proposed moral economy theory as a way of integrating discussions of economy and power into the anthropology of ethics. By weaving together moral anthropology and political economy, the book shows that ethical reflection does not float above structural realities. Activists' moral reasoning was deeply imbricated in their analysis of austerity, outsourcing and colonial legacies. In Thompson's (1991a) conceptualization of the moral economy, what was important was the obligations that developed between *groups* or *classes*, and how people used appeals to those obligations – rooted in particular ways of conceiving of the past – to contest contemporary changes in how goods and services were being exchanged.[1]

Economic anthropologist, Susana Narotzky (2016) is wary of moral anthropology, but also of the moralization of political protest. She worries that workplace and citizen campaigns based on injustice – rather than inequality – run the risk of not developing a broader understanding of the structural causes of the societal changes that they interpret as unjust. What is at stake here is the kind of consciousness that develops within the group, and the kinds of demands it makes. She writes:

> What is being fought for is a form of social worth that generally refers to a past moral covenant (Fordist–Keynesian) between capital and labour typical of Western core nations … They understand inequality in moral terms, that is, in terms of injustice. They seek redress, at best, in the form of a return to the 'status quo ante'. (2016: 86)

She continues:

> the understanding of inequality in terms of injustice traps most people within a moral rather than a politico-economic framework for mobilization, one which is not predicated on class, that is, on the awareness of the structural positions within the unequal ownership of the means to reproduce a livelihood. Therefore, the question is the following: can moral economy struggles become structural challenges to systemic social reproduction through praxis, as Thompson (1966) proposed for the making of the 'old' working-class consciousness? (2016: 87)

Certainly, the dangers she highlights resonate with what I found. Activists' vision of socialism was indeed a moral one, based on social ties and mutual responsibility rather than ownership of the means of production. But it was the use of theory from the anthropology of ethics that helped me to demonstrate the structural underpinnings of their vision. Moral critique did not trap NHS activists, nor did it fatally inhibit a structural understanding of the causes of inequality. Applying a modified version of Robbins' (2015) theory of the example helped me to develop the argument that the force of the NHS as an example of actually existing socialism derived from the fact that it was 'there', continuing to exist despite the onslaught of global capital. The NHS was an icon, but it was not just an icon. It was a publicly owned institution providing care based on a values discourse of free, universal and comprehensive services. State structures that intervened in society to facilitate the fulfilment of obligations to citizens not only should exist; they could and indeed *did* exist. Therefore, their removal would be wrong.

Battle lines were drawn around a particular imagination of the NHS *as* an example of socialism. Thus the interpretive battles over the meaning of the NHS, the obligations of the state and the nature of socialism were the basis of how groups formed. Just as artisans, peasants, keelmen and weavers allied with one another to protest the price of bread in the eighteenth century, retired and working healthcare professionals attempted to ally themselves with a wider public to protect the NHS in the twenty-first century.

It was the NHS that was able to bridge the gap between the particular interests of a small group, and the universal interests of a whole population. 'Universal' was written into the NHS core values: universal, free, comprehensive. There was a tension here between the NHS that was imagined and the NHS as it was; activists were aware that not everyone was able to access healthcare easily or equally (Pushkar, 2017; Kang, Tomkow and Farrington, 2019; Tomkow et al, 2020; Pushkar and Tomkow, 2025). But they continued to believe that the NHS could and should be truly universal, and that the people who contributed to making it less so were moral antagonists.

This book's contribution to debates on class centres on the morality at the heart of a possible class politics. I have pointed towards how, in the moral economy of NHS activism, different groups can cohere around a sense of shared interests with the values of the NHS at its core. Moreover, I have described how activists' ethics were entangled with how they conceived of their own interests. Sociologists (e.g. Zelizer, 2005) and anthropologists (e.g. Guyer, 1995) have repeatedly denaturalized people's own understandings of money, wealth and economy, thus destabilizing an objective view of class interests (Parry, 2020). Anthropological scholarship emphasizes the patient investigation required to work out how people perceive their interests in a particular social context at a particular time, and work towards achieving them.[2]

This book has demonstrated the ethical reflection, evaluation and work that goes into the affective and imaginative construction of material interests, as well as the consequences for social group cleavage and formation that follow from such social action. That is, describing interests as 'material' does not mean they are natural, determined or pre-given. They are open to interpretation that is the very stuff of what we might refer to as class consciousness. Activists understood the values of the NHS – universal, free, comprehensive – in such a way as to construct their interests as aligned not just with their fellow home-owning residents of affluent suburbs of Greater Manchester, nor with fellow holders of British passports, but with everyone in the UK. But they took their interpretation of the NHS into battle with people who understood the values of the NHS – and thus the boundaries of the community of interest – in different ways.

To put this in Marxian terms, I have brought out the development of a potential class-for-itself. Has this focus allowed me to elide the question of whether an alliance between NHS activists and a wider public genuinely constitutes a class-in-itself? Has my focus on the emic neglected the associated etic? Such an elision would be convenient, given the thorniness of the question of contemporary class (Carrier, 2015; Evans, 2023). In Thompson's view, the distinction between class-in-itself and class-for-itself was not so neat. Classes did not just make themselves through becoming 'aware' of a pre-existing social fact, of the nature of the base structure of society. People did not just *learn* that their interests aligned with other people's. The making of classes was an iterative process of becoming that developed through conflict, as people from different societal groups made their interests align through the forms of their struggles even as they became conscious of that alignment. In a well-worn quotation from a paper that formed part of his long-running dispute with Perry Anderson and structural Marxism, he argued:

> class is not this or that part of the machine, but the way the machine works once it is set in motion – not this interest and that interest, but the friction of interests – the movement itself, the heat, the thundering noise. Class is a social and cultural formation (often finding institutional expression) which cannot be defined abstractly, or in isolation, but only in terms of relationship with other classes; and, ultimately, the definition can only be made in the medium of time – that is, action and reaction, change and conflict. When we speak of a class we are thinking of a very loosely defined body of people who share the same congeries of interests, social experiences, traditions and value-system, who have a disposition to behave as a class, to define themselves in their actions and in their consciousness in relation to other groups of people in class ways. (Thompson, 1965: 357)

Actors, then, develop understandings of the groups that they are members of – classes – over time, *through* conflict with other groups. Crucial to this model is that the histories of these conflicts are made by the people involved themselves. They form understandings of who is in their group, who is in the group against which they are in conflict, and how their interests either converge or diverge through engagement in political contestation. I have not attempted to define NHS activists, clinicians, professionals or the people with whom they allied themselves in terms of their precise contribution to the reproduction of capitalist social relations. Instead I have shown how they were in conflict with other groups of actors, the defining of whom as moral antagonists was useful for activists in their activism, particularly in defining their own interests in ways that fostered broader coalitions, coalitions that may have the potential to disrupt or remake the state, society and capitalism.

As described throughout the book, the activist groups that I spent time with were not particularly diverse in their sociological make-up. In particular, Dunning KONP were mostly white, mostly retired and mostly fairly well off. Despite this lack of diversity among the activists themselves, they based their moral arguments on a sense of the public that extended broadly, transcending identities that included citizenship, ethnicity, age or, indeed, class. Scholars of class highlight the suspicion with which working-class people view middle-class morality, which they diagnose as moralizing, a process of class distinction in itself (Evans, 2006; Skeggs and Loveday, 2012). Where a class consciousness develops, it does so through a self-directed quest for respectability and dignity (Skeggs, 1997), rather than the humiliation of middle-class altruism (see also Todd, 2014).

The problem posed for my argument by such scholarship on class is that even if Dunning KONP activists might consider less wealthy people as allies and partners, even if their logic is based on equality and shared interests rather than charity and humanitarian compassion (Fassin, 2012), even if their moral and political arguments seek to dismantle rather than reinforce structures that perpetuate inequality, they are still middle class and would still be likely to be read as such by people who are not: as 'upper' (Evans, 2006: 33) or 'people on high money' (Balthazar, 2017: 222).

Therefore, the problem raised by evaluating my argument in the context of rigorous scholarship on class points both to the political challenge and to the scope for further scholarly investigation. If I – a hopeful activist – suggest the possibility of using NHS activism to build solidarity, then I – a careful scholar – must be willing to both accept the problems raised in the previous few paragraphs and to use them to generate new questions. How do migrants and working-class people who are not activists (or whose activism diverges from what I found in this project) understand the meaning of the NHS? Do they also understand cuts and privatization to be wrong, and if so, why? And, most importantly, if they do understand cuts and privatization to be wrong, then why are they not already in the activist groups I have described in this book? Is there a divergence on views on what the NHS is, was, or ought to be? In summary, what blockages might there be to the building of coalitions, and how might such blockages be overcome?

In Thompson's (1980) description of the development of working-class consciousness through the eighteenth and nineteenth centuries, all of the failures and impediments to the movements were lessons and memories that fed into the flourishing of radical egalitarian activity that emerged with Chartism. Although Chartism also failed to introduce a radically egalitarian society, he and others argued that the Chartists did at least have a mature sense of working-class consciousness as well as a willingness to express solidarity across classes (one source of their failure according to Stedman-Jones (1983)). It is possible that the setbacks of today will be remembered and serve the maturation of NHS activism, the consolidation of solidarity, as long as activists learn the right lessons.

I hope this book will serve not just as a scholarly examination of the moral economy of NHS activism in Greater Manchester, but also as a political intervention at a time when the meaning of the NHS is once again at the heart of everyday politics in England and the UK. By taking activists' ethical visions seriously, by tracing how moral arguments inform political alliances and by situating those arguments within structures of austerity and class, the book shows that moral economy is not a quaint historical concept but a living practice. The thundering noise of class struggle that Thompson described still echoes in contemporary battles over the NHS. Whether those battles coalesce into a broader movement for equality will depend on the capacity of activists, unions and parties to forge solidarities that live up to the universalist ideals they espouse. The NHS remains not just an institution that provides healthcare, but also a lens through which to imagine the good society.

Notes

Introduction

1 Scotland and Wales also have NHS organizations which are run separately. Northern Ireland has a Health and Social Care Service.

2 The Conservative Party and the Labour Party are the two largest political parties in the UK. The Conservative Party is also known as the Tory Party and I use both names interchangeably throughout the book.

3 The reader will note that I do not refer to a battle with the capitalists directly profiting from private healthcare. Activists did talk about private healthcare, as will become clear throughout the book, but I did not directly encounter private healthcare owners or administrators very often.

4 I have written about E. P. Thompson elsewhere (Pushkar, 2019), and parts of this section draw significantly on that work.

5 UK Uncut were an activist group that responded to the announcement of austerity budgets by raising awareness of businesses that they considered to be evading or avoiding payment of tax to the UK government (Sotirakopoulos and Rootes, 2014). Their actions began in 2010, with multiple well publicized protests throughout the early years of that decade.

6 In particular, Laidlaw (2014) and Robbins (2013) were critiqued by Kapferer and Gold (2018) and Ortner (2016). Laidlaw (2014) was exercised by Bourdieu's attempts to account for individual and social practices through reference to material conditions and unequal social relations between groups. Laidlaw saw Bourdieu's efforts (and Durkheim's legacy) as 'reductionist materialism' (Kapferer and Gold, 2018a: 13) to be avoided, thus leading Laidlaw to insufficient recognition of how the 'political and economic forces of history' (Kapferer and Gold, 2018a, 13) condition (and are conditioned by) the ethical judgements of people.

7 In some ways, that there ever was a debate seems bizarre. Anthropologists have long understood that people's ideas of who they are and how they should be are enacted in cultural contexts with material conditions (Munn, 1986; Graeber, 2001; Povinelli, 2011). See also Zelizer (2005) in sociology and Hyman and Brough in industrial relations (Hyman and Brough, 1975).

8 Activists, managers and politicians that I met used the words ethics and morality interchangeably. I do the same; I will not distinguish between morality and ethics. Instead, I will use both terms to refer to how actors evaluate things – including memories, events, actions, institutions, people, structures and aspirations – with regard to how things ought to be, or ought not to be, often using language that makes reference to what is good, bad, right or wrong. Underlying my decision to use the words interchangeably is a recognition that what is important for this book is the relationship between ethics/morality and politics rather than the distinction between ethics and morality.

9 For one anthropologist of ethics, Webb Keane (2016), politics is to do with the instrumental process of attempting to achieve (or mobilize towards) an end, whereas he defines the

ethical as 'an orientation to other people and activities that are undertaken for their own sake rather than instrumentally, as a means toward some further goal' (2019, 8). That is, ethics is about deciding what a person or group's ends should be. Politics is about figuring out how to go about achieving those ends. Thus he neatly brackets non-instrumental values from political instrumentality in a way that is inadequate to explain my ethnographic findings.

For my interlocutors the relationship between ethics and politics was not quite so clear-cut. Instead, actors' conceptualizations of what ends were possible within the means of the person – or the state – directly fed into what they considered to be right or wrong, good or bad. In Chapter 4 I will discuss how managers narrowed their ethical imaginations through reference to what was possible within the financial constraints that had been handed down to them. But activists contested the managers' ethical visions and the instrumental reasoning behind it. They sought to fight a political contest on moral grounds.

In a 2019 special issue of Anthropological Theory, editors Nancy Postero, Eli Elinoff, and Nicole Fabricant propose that politics should be understood as 'practices of world-making that proceed through the formulation of constellations of critique, disagreement, difference, and conflict'. This perspective highlights the role of ethnography in revealing how individuals and groups actively engage in shaping their social realities through everyday interactions and struggles. It is this latter definition of politics that this book follows. By politics I mean to refer to debate, argument and conflict regarding how societal and state structures and institutions are or should be organized. To politicize is to open to conflict and debate regarding causes and consequences. Importantly, the result of such debate will be the formation of new social ties and the breakage of old ones.

10 Thompson's privileging of experience has been criticized by historians for itself being under-theorized (Scott, 1991; Millard, 2020). On what basis could one historian claim to be able to access the authentic experience of the people she researches with more authority than another historian?

11 Thompson has been criticized (Anderson, 1980; Scott, 1991) for not taking account of the subtleties of difference in the various subjectivities lost within his description of a working class, and for a Romantic sweep that fails to ask just how universal a movement that foregrounds Englishness can be.

12 In the UK, a doctor is a 'junior doctor' from the point of finishing medical school, until they finish postgraduate training, that is, all doctors are junior doctors until they become consultant specialists or general practitioners. I am still a junior doctor and will remain so until at least 2027. In 2023, the BMA voted to change the term 'junior' to 'resident' doctor. Since my fieldwork took place before that change, I use the former term throughout the book, except Chapter 6.

13 Chapters 1 and 3 reflect further on how my positionality affected my analysis. I have also written elsewhere on 'how reflexive insight regarding the relationship between my positionality, my affect, and my behaviour led to important analytical breakthroughs with my interlocutors, particularly with regard to their own understandings of socialism and political alliances' (Pushkar, 2024: 46). In that paper, I argue for adopting an orientation of comradely critique (Slothuus, 2021) with regard to fellow activists. I have attempted to maintain such an orientation throughout this book.

14 Ethnographic fieldwork is necessarily partial, prioritizing depth over breadth (Mosse et al, 2023). I cannot claim that the activists with whom I spent time were representative of all activists campaigning against cuts and privatization in the NHS. Chapter 1 describes the demographics of Greater Manchester Keep Our NHS Public (KONP) in more detail: generally retired, white public sector professionals. My impression from attending

national meetings is that such demographics were common in campaigning organizations such as KONP and the Socialist Health Association. However, whether or not this profile was common among all NHS activists depends on how one defines an NHS activist. For example, there were also people working in the NHS who campaigned for better pay and working conditions, largely through their unions. Such people were often younger and from diverse backgrounds. As were those in organizations such as Medact, DocsNotCops and Patients Not Passports, which campaigned against healthcare charges for migrants. There was also significant overlap between all these different groups. On the other hand, there were also organizations who campaigned *in* the NHS on issues unrelated to cuts and privatization, such as the patient groups discussed in the *Thatcher and the market* section of Chapter 2.

[15] With managers, I benefited from having the confidence of an activist, Ronny, who was able to act as a gatekeeper for me. Ronny was a longstanding member of the Socialist Health Association. He features throughout the book, but I will describe him in most detail in Chapter 5. When I told him of my research project, he was fascinated and very keen to help. I sent him an email requesting support with finding managers to interview, aware that he knew many people from his activism and his work as a governor in several NHS trusts. He informed me that he had then forwarded my email to a database of over 100 people. Many people responded, and during the course of my fieldwork I did not manage to get around to interviewing all of them.

[16] This is not counting the activists who had previously held management positions in the NHS.

[17] The complex – and unfortunately unstable – ecology of NHS organizations is explained in Chapter 2.

[18] Councillors are the people elected to sit on local councils, which are the local governmental bodies in England. In Greater Manchester, there are ten councils. My interviews covered members of four of the councils, including three leaders.

[19] MPs are elected by British citizens to represent local constituencies in national government. All of the city of Manchester's MPs were Labour during the period of fieldwork. In Greater Manchester, there are 27 constituencies, 18 of which have Labour MPs and nine have Conservative MPs.

[20] Other groups occasionally mentioned in the book include Keep Our NHS Public, Health Campaigns Together, the Socialist Health Association, the British Medical Association, and Medact.

Greater Manchester KONP and Dunning KONP were affiliated to the national group: Keep Our NHS Public (KONP), of which I was also a member. KONP does not feature in the book much, except through Greater Manchester KONP and Dunning KONP's relations with it.

Health Campaigns Together (HCT) is an umbrella group that included KONP as well as many of the organizations affiliated to KONP. HCT took a leading role in organizing the biggest national protests, in concert with unions. Like KONP, HCT is on the peripheries of this book, only referred to through Greater Manchester KONP and Dunning KONP members' relations with it or attendance at events organized by it.

The Socialist Health Association (SHA) is a campaign group affiliated to the Labour Party. I discuss the SHA and two of its members, Ronny and Charles, in greater depth in Chapter 5. During my period of fieldwork, the previously dormant Greater Manchester branch of the SHA (GMSHA) was also reconstituted, allowing me to witness the interesting relationships between the various organizations and their members.

The British Medical Association (BMA) is the main trade union and professional association for doctors working in the UK. My involvement with the BMA was mostly before and after my ethnographic fieldwork. The BMA's relevance to NHS activism is discussed in Chapter 6, in an interview in 2025 with Dr Emma Runswick, deputy chair of BMA Council.

Medact is a national charity that campaigns for equality in global health and social justice. At the time of fieldwork, I was co-chair of the local chapter, Medact Manchester. We campaigned largely on issues relating to the health of forced migrants in Greater Manchester, and most specifically on the charging regulations introduced in the NHS by the Immigration Act 2014, discussed at greater length in Chapter 2. Medact is one of a number of organizations that have been campaigning against the charging regulations, including Doctors of the World and DocsNotCops.

Chapter 1

1 The Health and Social Care Bill became the Health and Social Care Act 2012, discussed at greater length in Chapter 2.

2 The question of how to improve the NHS is not one directly addressed by this book. Chris Thomas's (2022) book, which I engage with in more depth in Chapter 3, is a thoughtful take on what the NHS needs and how to get there.

3 The progressive media landscape may not have institutional power or hegemonic influence. But at least it exists now.

4 By 'we' I mean grassroots activists, not socialist intellectuals.

5 *The Guardian* reported that 40,000 people attended. KONP's own report cited 50,000 people.

6 He had discovered this by using the Labour Party's website, to which he directed me as well. I found that I was the 24,169,053rd baby born in the NHS.

7 See Chapter 5 for more on disagreements in Dunning KONP.

8 Tony (anonymized, like all other participants) died unexpectedly in 2018. Many of the other members of Dunning KONP and I attended the funeral. Leroy had worked with him for many years, and then remained close after retiring. We all continue to remember Tony fondly.

9 Although the Student Loans Company is incorporated as a private company, it is 'owned by the Secretary of State for Education, the Scottish Ministers, the Welsh Ministers and the Minister for the Economy in Northern Ireland. It is entirely government-funded and non-profit making' (Student Loans Company, no date). In 2018, in recognition that many people would never be able to repay their student loans, the Office for National Statistics reclassified the loans as partly genuine loans, and partly unrequited government expenditure (Moskalenko, 2020).

10 'Thatcher's children' is a quotation from Debbie, another member of Dunning KONP and Greater Manchester KONP, not Lily and Leroy. Debbie was referring to her younger siblings, both of whom are still working. Her brother was an anaesthetic consultant, and her sister was a midwife. Debbie, like Lily and Leroy, considered herself a child of the NHS and was using this description to contrast her ethicopolitical views on privatization with her siblings'. Both siblings worked in the NHS, but expressed deep misgivings about how it operated. They both *also* worked for private healthcare organizations.

11 Kenneth Clarke's own recollection of events is fairly similar to what Nancy described, as indicated in an interview published in 2021. He told his interviewer, the psychiatrist Peter Tyrer, that Margaret Thatcher believed the American insurance model was far superior to the NHS and had a complete plan to replace the tax-funded model with an insurance-based one. Clarke had to talk her down from the policy, which had been drawn up by his predecessor, John Moore. Moore was known as 'Mr Privatization' due to his involvement in the sell-off of other state services. After a period of illness, Moore lost his cabinet job and then lost his parliamentary seat. He then held directorships of

several multinational corporations. In 1992, Moore was elevated to the House of Lords as Baron Moore of Lower Marsh.

12 One key difference is that many of the Greater Manchester KONP members were already involved in contentious politics before retirement, and before the global financial crash. They had been active in their unions throughout their careers and thus considered that they had been NHS activists since the 1980s. I cover the longer history of Greater Manchester KONP's activism in Chapter 3.

13 See also Pushkar and Tomkow (2025).

14 Chapter 4 does explore differing interpretations of the NHS in more depth, in relation to managers and politicians.

Chapter 2

1 Cesar Abadia-Barrero (2022) documents something similar in his ethnography of healthcare workers resisting austerity in a Colombian hospital. Staff and patients get used to the environment crumbling around them and have to find ways to still provide healthcare with deteriorating equipment.

2 Most or all of their income was (and remains now) for NHS work. The initial GP contract cut and pasted many terms from the 1911 National Insurance Act. It required GPs to take 24/7, 365 days a year responsibility for patients, with penalties if not fulfilled. GPs also acted as 'gatekeepers' to specialist care, meaning that, except in emergencies, patients could only see a specialist if referred by their GP (Rosen, 2025). They were overseen by Executive Councils, with a capitation fee for each patient (Seaton, 2023).

3 The Windrush scandal is not discussed in this book for reasons of space. (For more information, see Gentleman, 2019; Stanley, 2022.)

4 Although recent academic studies have shed light on broader aspects of this relationship – such as colonial taxpayers paying for British welfare provision (Fitzgerald et al, 2020; Bhambra, 2022) – the essential insight that a higher standard of living in the metropole was dependent on colonial exploitation is hardly new. Walter Rodney's *How Europe Underdeveloped* Africa, was published in 1972. Even before that, in 1937 George Orwell wrote: 'the high standard of life we enjoy in England depends upon our keeping a tight hold on the Empire … in order that England may live in comparative comfort, a hundred million Indians must live on the verge of starvation – an evil state of affairs, but you acquiesce in it every time you step into a taxi or eat a plate of strawberries and cream.' He didn't explicitly cite the welfare state, but taxpayer-funded state institutions are of course one part of the 'comparative comfort' that he referred to.

5 Although, significantly, Conservative Secretary of State for Health, Keith Joseph, did hire US management consultancy firm McKinsey to advise on the 1974 NHS reorganization, thus setting a precedent for future interactions between the NHS and management consultants (Begley and Sheard, 2019).

6 Political scientist Ian Bruff's now classic paper on authoritarian neoliberalism (2014) documents how European governments' discourse on individual freedoms was increasingly undermined by the restrictive and coercive practices they employed to protect what they referred to as the 'free market'. The result was not a laissez-faire state, but a highly interventionist, authoritarian one, experienced as punitive by the most marginalized people (see also Koch, 2018).

7 Outsourced cleaning services have been associated with a poorer service (Lethbridge, 2012) and subsequent increase in infections among patients (Toffolutti et al, 2017).

8 One reason for low numbers initially was the persistence of the male breadwinner model, in which the men of the family did paid work outside the home. Unpaid care work was expected to be done by women in the household (Pedersen, 2018).

[9] Since then private provision has inexorably increased, despite evidence that quality of care is lower than that provided by the state or charities (Bach-Mortensen et al, 2024).

[10] Overseas recruitment of social care workers was banned in 2025. The status and stability of workers already in the UK was also undermined by plans announced by Home Secretary Shabana Mahmood to move towards an 'earned settlement' model for migrants, increasing the normal minimum period it takes for a migrant to be eligible for settled status from five years to ten years (Zhou et al, 2026).

[11] In 2000, Secretary of State for Health Alan Milburn consolidated this 'partnership' by signing a document entitled *For the Benefit of Patients: A Concordat with the Private and Voluntary Health Care Provider Sector.*

[12] The incentivization provides further evidence of Slobodian's (2018) point regarding how markets require active state intervention (see also Greer and Umney, 2022).

[13] Within Manchester, the largest provider trust, Manchester Universities NHS Foundation Trust, continues to pay for contracts dating from 1998 at Wythenshawe Hospital and 2004 at the Oxford Road campus in central Manchester. These payments totalled almost £80 million in the tax year 2023/2024 (approximately 3% of total expenditure) and the contracts run until 2033 and 2042 respectively (Manchester University NHS Foundation Trust Annual Report and Accounts 1st April 2023 to 31st March 2024).

[14] Both the Washington and Wall Street Consensus models were initially formulated to characterize developmental economics. The straight forward applicability of these models to the UK state speaks to the importance of finance in contemporary global capitalism (Adkins, Cooper and Konings, 2020; Christophers, 2023; Braun and Christophers, 2024).

[15] Ben Hunter (2025) has contrasted the morality of NHS trusts as profit-making organizations that export their services abroad while reliant on migrant labour with the ways in which 'overseas visitors' are treated unequally by the same NHS trusts.

[16] The revolving door between state, party political positions, private healthcare, lobbying firms and management consultancies continues to operate, as documented by journalists such as Peter Geoghegan (2024). Politicians and senior bureaucrats who have recently circulated between such appointments have included Patricia Hewitt, Simon Stevens, Alan Milburn, Dominic Cummings, Matthew Swindells, John Hutton, Norman Warner, Heather Iqbal, Mark Simmonds and Keir Cozens.

[17] Nevertheless, campaign groups and wider publics were not always taken in by such arguments. For example, the historian Colin Barker's (2010) paper describes the campaign to save Booth Hall Children's Hospital in North Manchester in the 1990s. The managers were tasked with selling the closure of the hospital to the restive local population. The managers put forward consultant paediatricians who argued their case predominantly on medical grounds. But the residents who were at the meetings responded with hostility, firstly pointing out contradictions in what the doctors said. More importantly, they admonished both the managers and the clinicians for believing that they knew better than the residents of areas whose hospital services were being withdrawn. The campaign was unsuccessful. Booth Hall Hospital closed in 2009. It was one of many closures across the country, leading to the steady decline of bed numbers examined in greater depth later in Chapter 2.

[18] I include more detail on these reforms than others before or after because this legislation was a key driver that galvanized many of the activists with whom I spent time. As described in Chapter 1, it was in response to the Health and Social Care Act that Galen and Iris organized a meeting that Lily and Leroy attended. The Dunning Keep our NHS Public group formed from that meeting.

[19] Criticisms at the time asserted that the Act would lead to fragmentation and duplication of services, that an inflated bureaucracy would increase cost, and that private providers

would 'cherry-pick' easy, simple services while neglecting complex but essential services, leaving non-profitable gaps to be filled by state services (Pushkar 2012). Professionals, managers and civil servants worried that the system envisaged by the Act was simply too complex to be the 'perfectly incentivized perpetual motion machine' (anonymous special adviser to David Cameron, quoted by Timmins 2018:12) that Lansley had in mind.

20 The government's Public Accounts Committee noted that 'the total deficit incurred during the franchise will be well above the level that Circle is contractually committed to cover, leaving the taxpayer to pick up the rest' (Public Accounts Committee, 2015). As Sam Freedman (2024) observes, this was a prime example of the state derisking a contract in order to incentivize private investment, with disastrous consequences that ultimately left the taxpayer footing the bill. Since then Circle, which is now owned by ADQ, the Abu Dhabi sovereign wealth fund, has grown to become England's largest network of private hospitals (Corporate Watch, 2024a).

21 Its abolition was announced in 2025.

22 The deal involved very little engagement from local councillors and MPs, much less the residents of Greater Manchester (Jenkins, 2015), who had rejected a mayor in a referendum in 2012.

23 There are 18 mentions of 'new models of care' in a 60-page document.

24 Charges apply to non-urgent secondary care and community services allied to primary care, including mental health, drug and alcohol, and community midwifery services. NHS trusts failing to comply with the new regulations face financial sanctions. This section draws extensively on a paper I wrote with Louise Tomkow (Pushkar and Tomkow, 2021).

25 I am referring not just to the Windrush scandal, which has been covered at length by Gentleman (2019), Stanley (2022) and Pushkar and Tomkow (2025), but also to wider restrictions that have not gained as much traction in national media (Kapadia et al, 2022).

26 This exact statement continues to be repeated by Conservative politicians (e.g. Hancock, 2019).

27 Please see also (Tomkow et al, 2020; Younis and Jadhav, 2020; Nazroo and Bécares, 2021; Essex et al, 2022; Kapadia et al, 2022; Lonergan, 2023; Worthing et al, 2023; Irons, 2024).

28 For example, a recent report from the conservative think tank, Policy Exchange, worries that the views of activist organizations that campaign against the hostile environment have been embedded into standard trust procedures, thus transforming 'public service – funded out of the hard-earned money of British taxpayers, for the benefit of British taxpayers' (Wolfson, 2025: 5) into a safe-haven, 'charity' or 'international aid organisation' (2025: 5).

29 I have explained elsewhere (Pushkar and Tomkow, 2025) why describing austerity as welfare retrenchment is more accurate, as it captures the classed differentiation in *which* aspects of state funding were reduced. In short, the services being cut were the ones more commonly used by the least well off. Wealthier people actually enjoyed a number of subsidies and tax cuts that have further entrenched inequality. O'Grady writes, 'The poorest 10% of working-age families have lost on average 20% of their net income since 2010 as a result of changes in welfare policy. The reforms have been linked directly to greater poverty, homelessness, indebtedness, and foodbank use' (2022: 1).

30 The rising cost of healthcare is a global phenomenon, the provenance of which continues to be a focus of academic debate (Rossen and Faroque, 2016; e.g. Atanda, Menclova and Reed, 2018). Much of the popular and media discussion of the cost of the NHS elides the fact that other countries are seeing the same problem, and instead seeks to blame increasing costs on a malevolent force, such as healthcare tourists or the feckless poor benefiting from moral hazard (Pushkar and Tomkow, 2025). That is, NHS spending provides another example of how the iconicity of the NHS has been put to use in welfare

nationalist narratives that interact with those put forward with the activists with whom I spent time.

31 This figure rose slightly after 2014, and significantly in 2019, when Prime Minister Theresa May announced a new funding settlement that raised the average annual real-terms increase back to 3.3% (National Audit Office, 2019).

When taking account of population growth, the slowing of funding increases is more remarkable. Average per-capita growth in spending for the whole period between 1949 and 2017 was 3.3%. Between 1996 and 2010 it was 5.4%. Between 2010 and 2017 it slowed to just 0.6%. But most other areas of state funding were also cut by the Tory government. The NHS was actually relatively protected in comparison to other services, especially local government (under whose budget most social care was paid for). Therefore, the *share* of government funds spent on the NHS rose after 2010. Between 1999 and 2010, health spending rose by 1.1% per year as a share of total public spending. Between 2010 and 2018 it rose by 2.1% per year (Charlesworth, Watt and Johnson, 2018).

32 Often such efficiencies translated to cuts of either services, staff or both. For example, both the 5 Year Forward View and Taking Charge spoke of a 'radical upgrade in prevention and public health' (Greater Manchester Combined Authority, 2015: 30) and 'investment in and expansion of prevention and integrated primary and community services' (Greater Manchester Combined Authority, 2015: 38). But public health and community services saw their funds restricted during this period (Buck, 2018; NHS Providers, 2018). Cuts to public health budgets were particularly criticized during the COVID-19 pandemic (Scally, Jacobson and Abbasi, 2020).

33 An article in the *Health Service Journal* reported: 'Operations are cancelled due to ageing ventilation systems and pipework, operating theatres are flooded, humidity and temperature regulation units cut out, pest infestations occur' (Tidman, 2024). A *Financial Times* article investigating why it was difficult to improve productivity in the NHS wrote:

> England had spent almost £37bn less than peer countries on health assets and infrastructure since the 2010s … Crumbling buildings meant services were disrupted at 13 hospitals a day in 2022–23 … The bill to repair NHS buildings and facilities rocketed to almost £14bn last month, compared with £11.6bn in the 2022–23 financial year, including £2.74bn worth of 'high-risk' repairs. (Hughes and Borrett, 2024)

In October 2024, the new Labour government announced an increase in NHS funding. Think tanks have noted that the £3.1bn earmarked for capital investment in health is dwarfed by a repairs backlog of £13.8bn. That is, the budget announced may just be enough to stand still, but not to improve and rebuild the NHS (Fisher, 2024).

34 Once the Conservative government understood that a lack of stocks was a problem it set up a 'VIP lane' to speed up procurement by avoiding open tendering processes (Dyer, 2022). Many referrals to the VIP lane came from Conservative politicians. Many of the companies who received PPE contracts were donors to the Conservative party (Wise, 2021). A judge later declared the VIP lane procurement process unlawful.

35 Leonora Merry and Sally Gainsbury (2023), analysts at the usually sober Nuffield Trust wrote:

> Our own work, and that of many others, has indicated that austerity was a contributing factor to declining resilience in the NHS in the years leading up to the pandemic, hampering its ability to manage the shock of Covid. Indeed, on 8 December 2016, three years to the day before the first Covid patient was hospitalised in Wuhan, we warned that 'slowing improvement in some areas of quality, combined with longer waiting times and ongoing

austerity, suggests the NHS is heading for serious problems. It seems likely that a system under such immense pressure will be unable, at some point, in some services, to provide care to the standards that patients and staff alike expect'.

36 NHS staff and their collective actions are the focus of Chapter 6. Staff had left due to burnout, bullying, excessive pressure, lack of job satisfaction and inadequate resources and equipment. One more key issue was pay suppression. Following the pandemic, the Tory government and then the new Labour government responded with recruitment drives, including of overseas staff. Another key strategy was recruiting people with less training, on lower pay, to do tasks that doctors and nurses used to do (Freedman, 2024; Greenhalgh and McKee, 2025).

37 New huge Nightingale hospitals were built to much media fanfare. However, they were unable to recruit enough staff to safely accommodate as many patients as they had space for (Christopher Thomas, 2022).

38 In response, hospitals raised admissions thresholds, in effect rationing care by admitting fewer patients. The reductions in admissions have been most pronounced in the most deprived areas, that is, the areas where people were already experiencing the worst structural insults to their health. As Cavallaro et al put it, 'It is not clear what has happened to more than half a million patients who would have been admitted for short emergency stays in 2019. Some are likely to have been treated elsewhere, potentially increasing the pressure on other services, while some are likely to have gone untreated' (2023). The other possibility that Cavallaro et al do not mention is that some of these people have resorted to self-paying for private healthcare.

39 Some people were on multiple pathways, so the number of unique patients was slightly less, at 6.3 million, but still close to one tenth of the UK population (NHS England, 2024a).

40 Since these new hospitals were, in effect, competing with NHS hospitals in both the self-pay and NHS markets, David Rowland, a researcher at the think tank the Centre for Health and the Public Interest, referred to private equity investment in the healthcare private sector as a 'bet against the NHS' (2022: 1). Rowland observed that the private sector invested over £2 billion in 40 new acute facilities in England between 2014 and 2022. Three private healthcare companies spent a further £1.1 billion on capital projects between 2016–2020.

41 The people availing of self-pay have not just been the wealthy. John Burn-Murdoch, data journalist at *The Financial Times*, reported that: 'The poorest now spend as much on private medical care as the richest, in relative terms. One in 14 of Britain's poorest households now incurs "catastrophic healthcare costs" in a typical year – where costs exceed 40 per cent of the capacity to pay' (2024). Whereas wealthier households were paying out-of-pocket, poorer households were often crowdfunding to afford these costs.

42 The source of his frustration is the healthcare activist focus on the sell-off, with inadequate focus on the buy-out. His research was not with activists, so he was unable to explore the provenance of fears of privatization, which is what I will do in Chapter 3. Nevertheless, Thomas does recognize that the sell-off is also taking place, even if it is bit by bit, rather than through a 'through a sudden, shock privatisation event' (Chris Thomas, 2022).

43 Mental healthcare is one area in which there has been a particularly prominent expansion in NHS funded care in privately provided organizations. The total independent sector mental health hospitals market was valued at £2.358 billion in 2023. It is estimated to have grown £296 million year-on-year, with the lack of NHS beds explicitly recognized as a key driver of this expansion (Gilburt, 2025).

44 All of the examples listed here are obvious, since anyone walking into hospital immediately sees the logo of the contractor company and the different uniforms of its staff. However,

there are also much less visible forms of ancillary service contracting, including information and communications technology. Companies such as Palantir and Infosys used the unique circumstances of the pandemic to gain a foothold in the NHS from which they have since expanded (Amin, 2023). These contracts are hidden behind commercial confidentiality but are thought to be getting longer and larger as time progresses (Corporate Watch, 2024b).

45 *The Financial Times* reports a higher number of 10% of elective care being provided by the private sector in 2024 (Hughes and Borrett, 2025).

46 The same paper reports an association between increased outsourcing and increased mortality from treatable causes. The direction of causation cannot be ascertained from that individual study. In a review paper by the same authors, they find that 'high rates of privatisation and outsourcing almost always corresponded with worse health outcomes in the studies' (Goodair and Reeves, 2024). Other research corroborates this finding (Borsa et al, 2023). Interestingly, some research indicates worse healthcare outcomes across the board, including in NHS hospitals, when more care is outsourced to private hospitals (Anderson et al, 2024).

One factor that politicians return to when advocating the use of the private sector is reduction of overall waiting lists by way of best use of available healthcare capacity. Wealthier people benefit most from this outsourcing, since it is wealthier people who are most likely to be 'cherry-picked' as easy patients who do not require the complex care that can only be provided in NHS hospitals (Kirkwood, Pollock and Roderick, 2024).

47 Each ICS includes a statutory integrated care partnership (ICP) and integrated care board (ICB). Together, they are tasked with commissioning and providing health and social care in defined geographical areas. They consist of NHS services, social care, and other organizations. The Hewitt review stated:

> The ICP is a statutory committee jointly formed between the ICB and the relevant local authorities within the ICS area. The ICP brings together the broad alliance of partners and is responsible for producing an integrated care strategy on how to meet the health and wellbeing needs of the population in the ICS area.
>
> The ICB is the statutory NHS organization responsible for bringing NHS and other partners together to plan and deliver integrated health and care services and accountable for the finances and performance of the local NHS as a whole.

The partnership model means that independent healthcare providers are no longer *just* providers. Theoretically, representatives of private companies could sit on ICBs, thus giving them a role in planning and commissioning local services as well.

Even as providers, private companies could potentially have more influence than previously. Providers now must join others to form provider collaboratives, with one provider appointed as lead in the collaborative, with the contract for coordinating with other providers and acting as main contact with the commissioners of services (Wickens, 2022). This lead provider could be an NHS or independent provider. For example, the provider collaborative for secure mental health services in Greater Manchester includes two NHS trusts (Greater Manchester Mental Health NHS Trust and Pennine Care NHS Foundation Trust) and two private companies (Cygnet and Elysium). Currently, the lead provider is Greater Manchester Mental Health NHS Trust, but nothing in the legislation mandates that it must be one of the NHS trusts rather than one of the private companies.

48 The plan describes a vision focused on three shifts: from hospital to community, from analogue to digital, and from sickness to prevention. It has been criticized for a lack of detail regarding the processes and structures that will be required to realize this vision,

particularly as its principles have been discussed by NHS policy makers and managers for many years (Cowper, 2025). Further given inadequate allocation of resources to achieve this bold vision, cost-cutting has repeatedly been prioritized.

49 Streeting has accepted donations from John Armitage (£95,000), Trevor Chinn (£13,500), Peter Hearn (£40,000 from him, £144,900 from companies controlled by him) and Jonathan Mendelsohn (£5,000), all of whom have financial interests in private healthcare companies (Colbert, 2024).

50 Streeting and Starmer's rationale is that every bit of healthcare capacity must be used to address the waiting list. One critique of this line of reasoning is that the key resource that the NHS is lacking is trained staff. Since the private sector does not contribute much to training, it does not actually add more resource, instead poaching staff from the NHS.

Chapter 3

1 This chapter focuses mostly on the activist perspective on privatization that I witnessed most commonly in Dunning KONP and Greater Manchester KONP, one that Ronny was mocking. Ronny's own perspective, which was less common among the activists with whom I did research, is explored more in Chapter 5.

2 When I use the term, 'moral fact', I do not mean that it is a fact that privatization is morally wrong. I mean to investigate the provenance of the observable social fact that activists consider privatization morally wrong. This way of using the term 'moral fact' is common in the anthropology of ethics and has a long history in scholarship going all the way back to Emile Durkheim and Marcel Mauss.

3 The word, temporality, is one often used by anthropologists (e.g. Munn, 1986; Bear, 2014) to refer to how people perceive, experience and engage with the passage of time. In a recent review of the sociological literature on temporality, Birgan Gokmenoglu (2022: 643) summarizes the political significance and necessity of considering how and why perceptions of time develop historically and vary socially and geographically:

> Time is as political as it is social. It is social because our understanding of the directionality of time, its measurement, allocation, and overall meaning is historically and geographically specific. That is to say, if we take advanced industrial countries of the West as an example, that time was not always understood as a linear and sequential progression of days, months, and years; it was not always measured by clocks and calendars; it was not always allocated according to the distinction between 'work' and 'life;' and time was not always money. Instead, these temporal structures and norms are the result of specific historical processes in specific contexts, like the transition to industrial capitalism or modernity and post-modernity. The temporal order of our lives is constructed and maintained by practices and structures of thought that only make sense as long as those practices and logics are collectively or inter-subjectively produced and reproduced. Time is political to the extent that those practices and logics are contested, negotiated, and reconfigured.

4 During my fieldwork, activists felt that in the past, commissioning had been chiefly vulnerable to privatization through contracting out services, for example, Commissioning Support Units that advised Clinical Commissioning Groups. However, the introduction of ACOs created a risk that the whole commissioning organization could be transferred to private ownership.

In December 2024, well after I completed fieldwork, I received an email from the Socialist Health Association that included the following definition of privatization. They acknowledged John Puntiss, Keep Our NHS Public, and the World Health Organization for the definition:

> A process in which non-governmental actors become increasingly involved in the financing and/or provision of healthcare services:
>
> - Franchising or contracting out to private, for profit, or not for profit providers;
> - Self-management, wherein providers are given autonomy to generate and spend resources;
> - Market liberalization or deregulation to actively promote growth of the private health sector through various incentive mechanisms;
> - Withdrawal from state provision, wherein the private sector grows rapidly as a result of a failure on the part of the government to meet the healthcare demands of the people.

The first two bullet points can be characterized according to Chris Thomas's (2022) formulation of the sell-off, whereas the latter two can be understood as the buy-out (both discussed in Chapter 2). At the time of my fieldwork, activists saw the final point as 'cuts' which led to a danger of privatization, rather than seeing it as itself privatization.

5 This was a minority view, even among the managers and politicians that I interviewed. Of course, my sample of managers and politicians was small and affected by selection bias in terms of who agreed to participate in the project. I think it is likely that in the wider population, many more managers and politicians may have held to this narrower definition of privatization, including within the Labour Party.

6 There have been multiple iterations of the GP contract since the inception of the NHS. But the basic structure of the model has remained largely unchanged.

7 NHS England plans had also discussed other 'new models of care', including ACSs (Accountable Care Systems). ACOs differed from ACSs in that ACOs were contractually integrated as a single organization, whereas ACSs could function as a 'loose alliance' of healthcare providers. In planning stages, ACOs and ACSs were both discussed as potential options by managers, politicians and activists in Greater Manchester. In this chapter, I only refer to ACOs, to aid readability.

The summary of the Health and Social Care Committee's report on ACOs (Health and Social Care Committee, 2018) had this to say about the variety of acronyms: 'understanding of these changes has been hampered by poor communication and a confusing acronym spaghetti of changing titles and terminology, poorly understood even by those working within the system. This has fuelled a climate of suspicion about the underlying purpose of the proposals and missed opportunities to build goodwill' (2018: 4).

8 Several similar names sprung up among a variety of campaigns after the success of the Hillsborough justice campaigners, who had encouraged people to support them using the hashtag #JFT96, meaning 'Justice for the 96' people who died. In 2016, a fresh inquest returned a verdict of unlawful killing, vindicating 27 years of campaigning by the victims' families.

9 The situation in Greater Manchester was complicated by Devo Manc and the existence of the Greater Manchester Health and Social Care Partnership (GMHSCP), which had already begun planning reforms before the announcement of STPs in the 5 Year Forward View. GMHSCP's plans involved LCOs (Local Care Organizations) rather than ACOs. (After the publication of the 5 Year Forward View, some boroughs, including Dunning, did include all of the available acronyms in their discussions: ACOs, ACSs, ICPs, LCOs, etc.) Although the acronym was different, the principle was the same: uniting the council with the CCG under a single body that would commission all health and social care

services. The first of Greater Manchester's LCOs was to be set up in central Manchester. Manchester's LCO was only for primary healthcare and social care, while secondary care would be provided by the already existing acute hospital trusts, to be merged under a single body called Manchester University Foundation Trust.

10 In the eyes of UK healthcare activists, the US is emblematic as evidence of the worst kind of private insurance coverage. They see it as inefficient, unnecessarily expensive, driven by profit rather than a desire for the welfare of the patient, and even corrupt. (E. P. Thompson shared this view, describing the American healthcare system as 'indecent', in contrast to the 'decent' NHS (Thompson, 1987)). Ethnographic studies have focused not just on how privatized healthcare is experienced by patients, but also how American insurance companies themselves work (Horton et al, 2014), corroborating activists' fears. These studies have uncovered a number of themes replicated in other countries where privatization is growing, such as cost-shifting and moral hazard (Dao and Mulligan, 2016). Other disciplines have corroborated these as well as other concerns, including overspending, informational asymmetry (Groce and Groce, 2020), market concentration and inadequate regulation (Bagley, 2015). Regardless, the clumping of all of these critiques together simply as 'Americanising' does set up a binary in which, at times, the goodness of the NHS has become implicitly (or even explicitly) linked to its Britishness. As described in Chapter 2, Andrew Seaton, citing multiple concrete examples, describes this process as 'welfare nationalism' (2023: 6).

11 Since John Lister was speaking at an open, publicly accessible conference, I have chosen not to anonymize him.

12 The most up to date figure at the time of writing, in summer 2025, is £2.16 billion spent by the NHS on purchasing private inpatient mental healthcare in 2023 (LaingBuisson, 2025). See *Privatization: the sell-off* section of Chapter 2 for more detailed exploration of NHS spending in the private sector.

13 Following the judicial review, these debates also extended beyond activists. In January 2018, an article in *BMA News* (Blackburn, 2018) referred to current reforms as 'the NHS being quietly reorganised' by 'quiet revolutionaries'. The article recognized the danger of whole ACOs being put out to tender, meaning 'the health needs of an entire population being managed by a profit-making company'. David Wrigley, a GP and member of BMA Council, well liked by many of the activists that I worked with, was quoted: 'There is a very genuine legitimate *worry* that services could be run by profit-hungry commercial organizations and that would be a serious *threat* to the founding values and ethos system of the NHS.' The article also quoted a patient representative from London, 'It feels a bit like following the US model – it's very *scary*'. I have added emphasis in both quotations to the emotions felt and the nature of the danger.

14 No managers or politicians that I spoke to used words as strong as 'fixed'. They told me that they did not expect Virgin or any other private company to sweep in to win the contract.

15 More background history on foundation trusts is described in Chapter 2.

16 The story of Circle in Cambridgeshire is recounted in Chapter 2.

17 Andrew Seaton (2023) cites a 1986 article in The Economist arguing that contractors had indeed stopped bidding for public sector contracts, in part due to union opposition creating 'administrative difficulties'. Krachler and Greer (2015) also agree with Catherine's view.

18 Although not often remembered by NHS staff, unions have a long history of opposition to private medicine in the NHS. As well as strikes to improve pay (e.g. by ancillary staff in 1973 and nurses in 1974), or to oppose outsourcing a service previously delivered in-house, such as cleaning services at various hospitals in the 1980s (Seaton, 2023), various unions voiced opposition to the existence of 'pay-beds' within NHS hospitals throughout the 1960s and 1970s, eventually leading to a Labour Party commitment to phase them out.

Importantly for an understanding of NHS employees' understandings of their interests – and their subsequent choices regarding political alliances – the doctors' union, the BMA, supported the existence of pay-beds. Therefore, in 1974, when Esther Brookstone, a union steward at Charing Cross Hospital, led a protest that shut down its pay-beds ward, the hospital's consultants stood opposed to the union's action. Despite the party's commitment, Labour governments in power from 1974 to 1979 did not eliminate pay beds. The subsequent Tory government halted progress on phasing them out. Instead, it negotiated a new contract with the BMA that allowed greater flexibility for consultants to undertake private practice as well as their NHS work. (Doctors' understandings of their own material interests, and the convergence thereof with societal interests under the aegis of the moral example of the NHS, is explored in more detail in Chapter 6.)

19 The latter has a chapter specifically on the benefits of removing a state monopoly in healthcare in order to increase competition and patient choice. It states, 'Our ambition should be to break down the barriers between private and public provision, in effect denationalizing the provision of health care in Britain' (2005: 78). Hunt is listed as one of the 23 authors, but it is not clear which authors contributed to each chapter.

20 A cursory look at the publications of think tanks that influence Tory policy – such as the Institute for Economic Affairs (IEA) and the Adam Smith Institute – shows up similar pro-privatization arguments. After Jeremy Hunt was promoted to Foreign Secretary in 2019, Matt Hancock took his place and activists pointed to the fact that the chair of the IEA had made significant donations to Matt Hancock's office. Activists described pro-privatization think tanks like the IEA as 'neoliberal', and considered that they were locked in a nexus that had grown to dominate political thought from Thatcher onwards, partly as a result of the 'revolving door' described in Chapter 2. In 2016, the IEA published a document entitled Universal Healthcare Without the NHS (Niemitz, 2016). It argued that CCGs already resembled insurers, and that their creation was one step towards creating a marketized system. The next step would be to give patients a choice as to which CCG to register with, and 'this market should also be opened to private non-profit and for-profit insurers. CCGs and non-NHS insurers should be free to offer a variety of health plans, including plans with co-payments and deductibles in exchange for rebates' (2016: xvi).

21 Importantly for this chapter, the historical narrative of pathways to privatization went back to Thatcher in the 1980s, but not further back to 1948 or earlier.

22 The NHS Confederation represents all organizations that commission or provide NHS services.

23 The view that privatization leads to worse care as a result of creating perverse incentives is one that is shared by many clinicians, bureaucrats and scholars (Chow, Ajaz and Priebe, 2019; Goodair and Reeves, 2024).

24 See Chapter 2 for more details on Circle.

25 Marx's own ethics, a subject of debate for many decades (e.g. Geras, 1984; 1992), have been explored in a recent book by philosopher Vanessa Wills (2024).

26 Keane uses his description of the 'surfaces of things' (2010: 68) to elaborate an understanding of how 'semiotic modalities' (2010: 68) inform moral reasoning. I include a full quotation here:

> By semiotic I mean this: people draw inferences about their circumstances on the basis of their perceptible experience of material forms, including the forms of language. Those inferences are not necessarily conventional – thus they do not treat things as 'symbols' – nor are they necessarily fully cognizable – thus they are not always 'interpretative' nor are the results necessarily 'meaningful'. Since material forms have causal sources, a semiotic approach is not to be confused with idealism or social constructionism. Since

> the inferences are usually informed by cultural knowledge, this approach is also not a pure phenomenology. (Keane, 2010: 68)

Thus the task for the scholar must be to acknowledge both the material phenomena being grasped in moral discourse *and also* the actors' perceptions of both the phenomena themselves and how their moral arguments might affect those phenomena. In sum, ethical arguments respond to – and consist in – people's perceptible experience of material forms, within which he includes language. His argument that people's inferences ought not to be understood as meaningful symbols or interpretations draws on his analysis of the Geertzian framework of culture as a text that can be observed, read and understood by the ethnographic fieldworker. Keane suggests greater complexity, since the people being observed are also doing their own interpretations, according to moral frameworks that may or may not be fully conscious, and are therefore not entirely transparent to an observer, although not entirely opaque either. I agree with Keane that meanings are slippery, in flux and not easy to grasp. But I hold onto the concept of interpretation, albeit cleaving more closely to Faye Ginsburg's version (1989), in which our interlocutors' interpretations are themselves the focus of moral and political struggle. Meanings are exactly what is at stake, with further stakes attached to the terms of battle. The task of the ethnographer, then, is to trace the stakes of the interpretive battle, and to map the consequences of the discourse and actions used in it. Concretely, in my case, why did activists interpret the NHS as a symbol of socialism, what did they mean by that interpretation, against what other interpretations did they mobilize theirs, with what consequences for social relations, institutional change and, moreover, for the interpretation itself?

[27] See note 79 in Chapter 2 for scholars who have examined the question of how privatization affects outcomes.

[28] The latter is contestable. It is not clear that private healthcare is superior to publicly provided healthcare. However, having access to immediate private healthcare is likely preferable to having to wait for public healthcare.

[29] This was a normative belief rather than a descriptive statement. In other words, universality was an NHS value that activists held to. Therefore, they objected if they felt it was being undermined. Members of Dunning KONP and Greater Manchester KONP were very aware of the fact that issues of access to NHS care were worsening (Potter et al, 2017; Kang, Tomkow and Farrington, 2019; Tomkow et al, 2020) during the period of fieldwork, and keen to join up with campaigning groups that sought to address these issues, including DocsNotCops and Medact (see also Pushkar and Tomkow, 2025).

[30] Sociologists of labour, Ian Greer and Charles Umney (2022), recently explored the relationship between marketization and workers' employment conditions for workers. I quote from a book review in a socialist newspaper:

> Although orthodox economics suggests that competition threatens profits, the authors argue that competitive markets nonetheless remain beneficial to capitalists as a 'disciplinary' tool to control labour through low-paid, insecure jobs that keep the labour force compliant, and to reduce political oversight by enabling capitalists to make decisions unilaterally. In short, Greer and Umney state baldly: 'Marketisation disciplines workers and subverts democracy'. (O'Toole, 2023)

[31] In central Manchester, addiction services have been provided by a few different charities including RISE, and now Change Grow Live. Early Intervention Services, which assess and manage people during and following a first episode of psychosis, were briefly provided by Rotherham Doncaster and South Humber NHS Trust, but has been brought back in house now.

[32] Labour scholars have explored this vulnerability. For example, Beverly Silver (2003: 4) has written of how the hypermobility of contemporary global capital has created a race to the bottom for states competing for private investment.

[33] Private cataract surgery provides a useful example within the NHS. A recent report from the Centre for Health and the Public Interest (Rowland, 2025) found increasing provision by private companies despite there not being any publicly stated aim from NHS bureaucrats to contract out. Instead, the private sector looked for – and found – a route to accessing state funds:

> Between 2019 and January 2025 there have been over 130 new eye care clinics set up in England, and the volume of NHS cataracts being delivered by private companies has increased by 400%.
>
> But, we have not seen any clear plan by NHS England or local Integrated Care Boards (ICBs) to increase capacity in the private sector to this degree. We found very few contracts for work by the private sector being put out for tender by the NHS, which is what usually happens when private companies are brought into to deliver NHS care.
>
> Instead, we found that private companies have been making use of the very weak regulations governing the NHS market. These rules allow companies to set up clinics which are capable of delivering NHS cataract care to the required standard and to then demand a contract from the local ICB to treat NHS patients.
>
> As a result, over the past 6 years private companies have been setting up clinics in parts of the country even though the ICB had not identified a need for them.

[34] In a recent interview, the outgoing head of NHS England, Amanda Pritchard, made exactly this point. The interviewer quotes: 'in the case of NHS capital spending, relying entirely on state largesse "hasn't worked for the last 15 years or so". Private investment is needed to help plug the gap, she says' (Neville, 2025).

[35] Hood and Dixon define NPM as 'a set of loosely related ideas about government and public service reform … ostensibly intended to create "a government that works better and costs less"' (Hood and Dixon, 2015:265), often summarized by the aphorism: 'what matters is what works'. NPM seeks to produce more effective and efficient public services by way of combining top-down reorganization and surveillance with organizational downsizing and decentralization (Ferlie et al, 1996). Since it has often resulted in the privatization of public services, NPM has been described as a 'market-based ideology' (Ferlie et al, 1996: 9).

[36] The figure of 500,000 is from Chris Thomas's book (2022). However, the organization has continued to expand since Thomas's book was published. At the time of writing, in May 2025, the Operose website states it provides primary care for 700,000 people across 82 locations.

[37] One way of conceptualizing this concession might be as a class compromise. Gabriel Winant (2021) uses this term to analyse the working-class acceptance of privatized healthcare in postwar US, as long they were insured through their work. Unions calculated that health insurance for employees was as much as they could achieve. It was a compromise insofar as it did not guarantee comprehensive or universal healthcare, particularly for those who fell out of work. It also consolidated a male breadwinner model, since women and children were only eligible for healthcare through the largely male steel workers' employment. Winant's study follows the development of healthcare through the decline of the steel industry, when many more workers lost their jobs. The power of Winant's study lies in following not just the material effects of the decline of

steel, but also the cultural and institutional deposits laid by the initial class compromise, and how they contributed to opening and closing political possibilities in later years. Steel workers' decades of work contributed to their own ill health, while their partners and daughters took on professional caring roles in the expanding health industry.

Chapter 4

1 This chapter draws heavily on a paper published in the *Cambridge Journal of Anthropology* (Pushkar, 2023).

2 See also Appadurai (2012), who takes a different tack, but holds to the contemporary importance of numerical calculation.

3 Theresa May said this to a nurse who had not had a pay rise for eight years and was having to use food banks to survive. A clip of the interchange subsequently went viral, and these words became part of British political lexicon. It was repeated to me many times during fieldwork, earnestly by managers and sarcastically by activists.

4 See also, Strathern on a 'tyranny of transparency' (2000c: 309), cf. Piliavsky (2013).

5 Umney and Greer argue that the disciplinary effects on people's subjectivities were not the only effects of the coeval processes of audit and marketization:

> Followers of Michel Foucault make an important point when they emphasize that in a 'neoliberal' society, market competition plays a central role in structuring everyday life. Whether people are successful in the market or whether markets function as advertised matters less for them than the point that subjectivity changes. Our interviewees in French hospitals spoke of 'privatization of the spirit' to describe how their working patterns were changing ... However, this language would seem to downplay the problem. A job seeker forced to choose between accepting a low-wage job and losing unemployment benefits; a nurse who will not receive a pay increase because her workplace has been outsourced or privatized; and a musician advised by his digitalized agent to advertise a lower fee: all these individuals would be lucky to experience marketization only in spirit. Marketization cannot be understood separately from the power relations between classes that determine it and the distribution of wealth and income that result from it. (Greer and Umney, 2022: 156)

Whittle et al (2024) and Armstrong (2024) have also written regarding the effects of audit cultures on NHS patient care within psychiatric institutions.

6 See Chapter 2 for more detail on the Health and Social Care Act, NHS England, foundation trusts and clinical commissioning groups, and Chapter 3 for more detail on Accountable Care Organisations, Accountable Care Systems, Local Care Organisations, Integrated Care Partnerships and Integrated Care Systems.

7 It is worth underlining that the NHS and NHS England are not the same thing. NHS England was set up by the Health and Social Care Act 2012 to run the NHS *in* England. The subsequent Health and Care Act 2022 has illustrated a pendulum swing by making further changes. The 2022 Act gives back to the Secretary of State for Health and Social Care more power to intervene directly in local healthcare administration.

8 The dynamic complexity of the NHS making it difficult for local politicians to scrutinize it continues to be a problem (e.g. Dulhanty, 2022).

9 That interview took place in April 2018. At the time of writing, in summer 2025, Greater Manchester trusts are in severe financial difficulty. The Shanley Report (NHS England, 2024b), which investigated malpractice in Greater Manchester Mental Health Trust in 2022, stated that the Greater Manchester Integrated Care Board (ICB) reported a deficit

of £125m after the first four months of 2023/24. Rather than recognition that 'overspend' may be a symptom of an inadequate budget, NHS England instead reprimanded the ICB, placing it in the 'mandated support' category of NHS England's regulatory regime (Anderson, 2024).

10 See Chapter 2 for more on the four-hour target.

11 Wilson (2012, 2015) has argued that the histories of British bioethics and medical accountability are themselves inextricable from the histories of Thatcher and neoliberalism in the UK.

12 That is not to say that Julian's savings gave him complete freedom. He told me that part of a manager's role was to contribute to corporate strategy. But once the organization had decided its plan, the manager ought to stick to it most of the time, even if he had been advocating for something different to what was eventually chosen. The times when Julian felt compelled to speak out against the council's actions had been exceptions that he could count on his hands. Moreover, when I asked if he could tell me more about them in our interview, he said no. Although he had spoken out in those incidents, he had not spoken out willy-nilly. He had chosen particular ways to make his voice heard in order to effect a change in direction that complied with his own understanding of his and the council's moral obligations. Telling me more about them in 2018 would not have been a useful way to address those past conflicts and so he remained quiet.

13 Julian, Olga, Nancy and Betty all felt the pressure to make changes that reduced cost. Such pressure was clearly onerous and difficult to resist, fitting with the disciplinary power of audit technologies as described by Shore and Wright (2015). And yet, in these managers' own moral reasoning, there were good reasons to over-ride that pressure. They had ideas that had to be enclosed and debates foreclosed in order for them to comply. Julian, Olga and Nancy found ways to not allow these debates to be foreclosed. Audit could not quite be as totalizing as its proponents may have liked. Other forces were required to augment, facilitate or create space for audit.

In the *Accountability as transparency* section, I discussed the inability of activists to find out which services had been or were going to be cut or privatized. Activists also described their frustration with councillors who openly admitted to not understanding the structure of the NHS. Activists were thus unable to hold people accountable for changes to the NHS, since the changes were not visible to them. The changes were hidden and thus illegible. Strathern (1997) discussed how one of the aims of audit was precisely to make organizations legible. The legibility she described was according to a particular model, thus facilitating the use of measures to describe the degree to which the organization fitted a pre-set ideal. Where an organization did not fit the model, auditors did not attempt to understand what the organization actually did; how it did, in fact, work. Instead, the lack of fit between the auditors' findings and the audit technology's model led the auditors to conclude that the organization was 'somehow ... not there' (1997: 9). While she found the lack of curiousity allowed within audit 'extraordinary' (1997: 9), she also found a potential sanctuary for creativity. Perhaps if auditors weren't looking – or, rather, were unable to see – then academics and other professionals could let their ideas run free.

But illegibility has a different function in this chapter, in which activists were not auditing bureaucrats, but utilizing other forms of accountability. Activists were attempting to render managers' and politicians' actions transparent and hold them answerable for those actions. Unlike auditors, activists were far from incurious regarding what the organizations were doing and how they were going about it. However, activists were actively blocked from learning about service retrenchment and its consequences. Whom did this illegibility protect? Strathern wondered if the illegibility (to audit) of some professional activities might afford scholars freedom to act in line with motivations other than those measured by auditors. However, I found that in NHS transformations, the mish-mash of accountabilities and professional or moral codes was different. Rather than protecting the creative professional from the diktats of auditing managers, illegibility protected the manager from the morally enervated activist. Illegibility was one way in which debate regarding appropriateness or goodness of reforms was foreclosed. Thus the manager could get on with counting beans and reforming services within the enclosed limits of the available beans.

However, Betty, Julian, Nancy and Olga did not simply get on with counting beans. Upwards accountability was partially blocked, shielding bureaucrats from political challenge, foreclosing debate. As such, Betty and Julian were aware of activist discourse but had only had occasional meetings with them. But managers and politicians were moral agents themselves. They were accountable to their own consciences and internalized ethical codes. At times they reasoned that despite fulfilling an obligation to spend within one's means, the transformations they were administering were failing on other obligations that they considered at least as important, such as to provide universal, free and comprehensive healthcare to all. Therefore, the enclosure of conceptualizations of what could be achieved was broken, occasionally leading to an openness to debate. Julian broke open the foreclosure of political debate through his own moral reasoning.

It is this combination of enclosure and foreclosure that I have described as ideological closure in this chapter. It was closure – with the appearance of a debate that had already been settled and could not be reopened – that so enervated activists, who were attempting to prise it open.

Chapter 5

1 Other writers and scholars (Seymour, 2016; Nunns, 2018; Manwaring and Smith, 2020) have documented the unique social and political factors that led to his victory. Rather than recount that story, I merely note that his election represented a break from the recent history of the party.

2 Ed Miliband is the son of Ralph Miliband, who will be discussed later in the chapter. They do not share the same political views.

3 Smith (2012) and Evans's (2017) work focuses on predominantly white communities.

4 Graeber's (2014) discussion of the PMC leaves the Ehrenreichs' theorization mostly intact. His innovation was to apply it to universities, especially academic anthropologists. He combined his analysis with a discussion of the financialization of universities, drawing links between neoliberalism and what he understood as the toothlessness of 'vulgar Foucauldianism' (2014: 43) and its critiques of contemporary politics. Graeber's provocation can be summarized thus: by concentrating their intellectual perspicacity on post-modern critique, scholars had acquiesced to the expansion of neoliberal management techniques through the university. Moreover, academics had not just allowed the PMC to take over; they were members of the PMC. Cowan's (2014) response to Graeber noted the value of his essay as a polemic but wondered about the elisions he had made to advance his argument. In response to his accusation that academics had not resisted the advance of NPM and audit cultures through the university, she wondered where he had been for the past decade. She finds Graeber's analysis 'much too smooth' (Cowan, 2014: 91), citing multiple examples of exactly the kinds of resistance that he denied the existence of.

5 There is a symmetry here with Winant's (2019) description of American activists' use of PMC in recent years. In my interview with Maxine, she told me she had also been called a Blairite, and was keen to clarify that she was not one. She found the reductive

binary – socialist or Blairite – simplistic and frustrating, failing to account for any kind of nuance.

6 Her argument was similar to that of Hilary Wainwright, a scholar-activist who had been associated with the New Left in the 1980s. Wainwright (2015) was among the influential voices that endorsed Corbyn's leadership campaign, writing that 'Jeremy Corbyn should be supported not as an attempt to "reclaim the Labour Party" but as a transition to a political organization beyond the Labour Party and beyond parliamentary politics'.

7 The party is often referred to as a broad church. The term is meant to refer to a wide array of political views that can co-exist while working together within one ecumenical party.

8 Labour Party members are organized according to constituencies, with each constituency further broken down to branches. Typically, branches and constituencies meet monthly to discuss local and national political issues. Motions can be brought and voted on, which are considered to influence local and national policy.

9 Describing Momentum as 'pro-Corbyn' is somewhat simplistic. Its own website states, 'Momentum is a people-powered, vibrant movement. We aim to transform the Labour Party, our communities and Britain in the interests of the many, not the few.' However, in practice, many of its members, as well as its detractors, did describe Momentum as pro-Corbyn while he was Leader, as they saw him as the Leader most likely to help Labour members to achieve these aims. Lewis Bassett's doctoral thesis (2020: 175), based on empirical research undertaken at the same time as mine, argued that Momentum 'initially sought to build "grassroots power", [but] the organization instead developed into one most concerned with helping Corbyn win his intra-party battles as well as helping Labour compete in general elections'.

10 The cabinet is the senior decision-making body of the council. Dunning Council's website states: 'It is responsible for the strategic management of Council services, and consists of a Cabinet Leader and 7 other Cabinet Members, each of whom holds a Portfolio covering a particular service area.'

11 Nairn counted five million members (1964a), although Anderson did point out that they were not all working class, and that many working class people did support the Tories (Davis, 2003).

12 A section of his paper carries the memorable title: 'From New Left to new Labourism' (Bassett, 2019: 4).

13 The Nairn-Anderson theses have also been criticized for not explaining the fact of social democratic parties failing to usher in socialism *anywhere*. As well, it has been noted that the alliance between the bourgeois and the aristocracy was not a British peculiarity, but an international phenomenon (Haider, 2016).

14 In 1981, it changed its name to the Socialist Health Association, to signify its members' belief that preventive measures to improve health were more important than healthcare itself.

15 Ronny was aware of the mistrust from some quarters, and the labels that were attached to him. He told me that the people who mistrusted him probably thought they disagreed with him, but they might not disagree with him if they actually spoke to him. Later, he described conversations that he had had with members of KONP and its affiliated organizations in which he clearly did disagree with them on the role of private companies and third-sector organizations in the NHS. He felt that since GPs had always been independent contractors, the private sector had effectively always had a role in the NHS, and that this fact undermined arguments against privatization. Moreover, he argued that KONP members lacked knowledge regarding how the NHS ran in practice, and that their fears regarding privatization were unfounded.

16 Whenever I asked Ronny whether he was a Blairite, or what Blairism might mean, he steered the conversation towards other areas, such as Tony Blair's dislike for the word, 'socialism', meaning that under New Labour it had become toxic. Given Ronny's loquacity, I usually forgot to come back to the question until the next time I saw him, when the same thing would happen again. In short, I never got a straight answer to the question of whether he was a Blairite or a socialist, and I never heard him describe himself as either.

17 For Labour Party conference 2017, the SHA had submitted a motion on the NHS that was passed unanimously, and that got a lot of attention from NHS activists. The motion, Composite Motion 8, called for Labour to halt and reverse plans for Sustainability and Transformation Plans and Accountable Care Organizations, to reverse privatization and to increase funding in order to achieve 'an NHS that is publicly owned, funded, provided and accountable'. At the SHA meeting in November, several members congratulated Charles for his role in writing and promoting the motion, phrasing their congratulations as 'returning the NHS back to being socialist'.

18 In 2015 there were 672 members. In 2016, there were 683.

19 Afterwards, Ronny wrote on Facebook, '*As expected*, the officers of the SHA have decided to sack me'. I note two points here. First, I have added italics to emphasize what he later confirmed to me: that he had always suspected that Charles and others were trying to squeeze him out of the SHA, because they thought he was a Blairite. Second, he was actually not dismissed by the officers. He was dismissed by a tribunal that found that he had broken some of the SHA's rules. (I refrain from giving further details regarding the rules he was found to have broken.)

20 He told me that others shared the view that he had been pushed out, including people associated with the aforementioned Manchester MP. He even wondered if the conspiracy had included involving the staff members of an outside organization in baiting him to commit one of the breaches. When he told me this, I must have raised an eyebrow, as it seemed somewhat far-fetched to me. He added that a friend, John, had suggested the theory, and that John was 'a bit of a conspiracy theorist'. He added, 'Well I don't know, I find it a bit hard to believe that it's a conspiracy. But it might be.' It might be. Although some of these theories seemed outlandish to me, I have no way of knowing if they were true.

Chapter 6

1 Agenda for Change does not apply to outsourced services, hence the incentive for trusts to contract services not just to private companies but also to wholly owned subsidiary companies, whose employees would not benefit from the national collective pay bargaining institutionalized through Agenda for Change.

2 In 2023, the BMA voted to change the term 'junior' to 'resident' doctor. Since my fieldwork was before the change, the book mostly refers to junior doctors. In the interview, Emma and I interchange between the two terms. The BMA's press release on changing the term reads: 'Resident doctors are fully qualified doctors who are either currently in postgraduate training or gaining experience as locally employed doctors, to become the consultants, GPs or specialists of tomorrow. They form the largest single group in the UK's medical workforce, with many having more than a decade of experience as highly qualified professionals.' https://www.bma.org.uk/bma-media-centre/junior-doctors-change-name-to-resident-doctors

3 See Chapters 2 and 3, including note 102.

4 BMA council is the principal executive committee of the trade union.

5 Doctors Vote and Broad Left are internal groups, made up of BMA members, who seek to exert pressure on the BMA as a whole. Emma Runswick and I are members of Broad

Left, more information on which can be found here: https://www.doctorsbroadleft.com/ More information on DoctorsVote can be found here: https://doctorsvote.org/

6 SAS is an abbreviation for Specialty, Associate Specialist and Specialist. The term refers to doctors with significant postgraduate experience who are neither consultants nor on a training contract.

7 For more on the history of the BMA see Seaton (2023) and Watkins (1987). For more on Whitley Councils see NHS Employers (2025).

8 Jeremy Hunt was Secretary of State for Health and Social Care. See Pushkar (2019) for background on that strike.

9 Multiple laws have been passed from 1980 onwards making it more difficult to take industrial action (Daniels, 2023). For example, under these laws, strike ballots must be conducted by post, meaning that unions and members must invest in having correct information including home addresses. In addition, the Trade Union Act 2016 stipulated that, for strike action to be valid, there had to be at least 50% turnout.

10 In 2021, there 69,691 doctors in the UK, 13,035 of whom had not trained in the UK. The General Medical Council stated that increases in numbers of doctors was increasingly being driven by international medical graduates (General Medical Council, 2022).

11 For people living in the UK with a visa, absence from work for ten consecutive working days would require the employer to notify the Home Office.

12 See Greenhalgh and McKee (2025) for background on physician associates.

13 Following an inquest or investigation into a death, a coroner may issue a Regulation 28 Prevent Future Deaths (PFD) report to a person or institution, where the coroner believes that action to address some of the identified concerns should be taken to prevent future deaths.

14 Waiting list initiatives are extra clinics and operating lists put on by NHS trusts to clear backlogs. The professionals working for these initiatives are usually internal employees who are paid higher rates for working extra-contractual hours, for example, in the evening or at the weekend.

15 Emma is referring to reinforced autoclaved aerated concrete (RAAC). RAAC is a lightweight form of precast concrete, frequently used in public sector buildings in the UK from the mid-1950s to the mid-1990s. RAAC has a lifespan of 30 years. As such, buildings made with RAAC are now beyond its lifespan and at risk of collapse. The Department for Health and Social Care says there are 54 hospitals that contain RAAC and that '7 RAAC-affected hospitals will be replaced by 2030 through the New Hospital Programme; and that we remain committed to eradicating from the NHS estate entirely by 2035' (DHSC Media Team, 2024).

16 Foundation Year 1 is the first year of work for doctors following graduation from medical school.

17 From April 2025, the national living wage is £12.21 per hour, which equates to £25,396 for people working 40 hours per week. The basic salary for a Foundation Year 1 doctor is £36,616 for a doctor working 40 hours per week.

18 This quotation from Bevan has actually been attributed to Trevor Griffith's television play, *Food for Ravens* (1997).

Conclusion

1 But, as Palomera and Vetta (2016) have decried, moral economy theory has not always been used in this way. Moral economy theory has been criticized for the heterogeneous ways in which the two words have been used, leading to Didier Fassin describing the concept as 'trivialized' and Chris Hann describing it as 'muddled' (both quoted by Carrier, 2018: 18). Carrier's (2018) valiant attempt to clarify the discussion by providing a more

precise definition focuses on reciprocal obligations that develop within relationships between individuals. Palomera and Vetta (2016) have been among those calling for a return to something closer to Thompson's theorization. They note how much recent anthropology uses moral economy as a foil to discuss contemporary political economy, in whose cracks and crevices solidary networks of exchange continue to exist that are labelled as moral economies. Thus the two types of economy are seen as separate entities, moral economy is opposed to political economy in a manner akin to Polanyi's (2001) separation of embedded and disembedded economies. As Palomera and Vetta (2016) argue, such an approach misses Thompson's point somewhat; they maintain that all economies are simultaneously political *and* moral.

2 Even Vivek Chibber (2022), sometimes critiqued as a class reductionist or class abstractionist (McCarthy and Desan, 2023) recognizes that interests are constituted in, by and through culture and ideology. As Lorelei Jones, medical anthropologist, and Kirsten Armit, health services researcher, put it recently in a paper on doctors in senior management positions in the NHS, 'Interests are shaped by meaning and meanings may be used to promote interests' (2025: 2).

References

Abadía, C. (2022) *Health in Ruins: The Capitalist Destruction of Medical Care at a Colombian Maternity Hospital*. Durham, NC: Duke University Press.

Abram, S. (2017) 'Contradiction in contemporary political life: meeting bureaucracy in Norwegian municipal government', *Journal of the Royal Anthropological Institute*, 23. doi: 10.1111/1467-9655.12592.

Adkins, L., Cooper, M. and Konings, M. (2020) *The Asset Economy*. London: Polity Press.

Allinson, I. (2022) *Workers Can Win: A Guide to Organising at Work*. London: Pluto Press.

Amin, L. (2023) *Exclusive: NHS hospitals told to share patient data with US 'spy-tech' firm, openDemocracy*. Available at: https://www.opendemocracy.net/en/palantir-peter-thiel-nhs-england-foundry-faster-data-flows/ (Accessed: 12 March 2025).

Anderson, H. (2024) *Consultants sent in to tackle overspending at nine ICSs, Health Service Journal*. Available at: https://www.hsj.co.uk/finance-and-efficiency/consultants-sent-in-to-tackle-overspending-at-nine-icss/7037483.article (Accessed: 3 June 2025).

Anderson, M., Friebel, R., Maynou, L., Kyriopoulos, I., McGuire, A. and Mossialos, E. (2024) 'Patient outcomes, efficiency, and adverse events for elective hip and knee replacement in private and NHS hospitals: a population-based cohort study in England', *The Lancet Regional Health – Europe*. The Author(s), 40: 100904. doi: 10.1016/j.lanepe.2024.100904.

Anderson, P. (1964) 'Origins of the present crisis', *New Left Review*, 23.

Anderson, P. (1980) *Arguments within English Marxism*. London: Verso.

Anderson, P. (2020) 'Ukania Perpetua?', *New Left Review*, 125(Sept/Oct). Available at: https://newleftreview.org/issues/ii125/articles/perry-anderson-ukania-perpetua. (Accessed: 26 November 2020).

Appadurai, A. (2012) 'The spirit of calculation', *The Cambridge Journal of Anthropology*, 30(1): 1–17. doi: 10.3167/ca.2012.300102.

Armstrong, N. (2024) *Collaborative Ethnographic Working in Mental Health: Knowledge, Power and Hope in an Age of Bureaucratic Accountability*. Abingdon: Routledge.

Atanda, A., Menclova, A. K. and Reed, W. R. (2018) 'Is health care infected by Baumol's cost disease? Test of a new model', *Health Economics (United Kingdom)*, 27(5): 832–849. doi: 10.1002/hec.3641.

Axelsson, R. (2000) 'The organizational pendulum: healthcare management in Sweden 1865–1998', *Scandinavian Journal of Public Health*, 28(1): 47–53.

Bach-Mortensen, A., Goodair, B., Esposti, M., Walker, C. and Barlow, J. (2024) *Evidencing the Outsourcing of Social Care Provision in England.* Oxford: Nuffield Foundation.

Bagley, N. (2015) 'Medicine as a public calling', *Michigan Law Review*, 114(1): 57–106.

Bale, T. (2016) 'The loser takes it all. Labour and Jeremy Corbyn: a response to Steve Richards', *The Political Quarterly*, 87(1): 18–19.

Balthazar, A. C. (2017) 'Made in Britain: Brexit, teacups, and the materiality of the nation', *American Ethnologist*, 44(2): 220–224. doi: 10.1111/amet.12471.

Barker, C. (2010) 'Ideology, Discourse and Moral Economy: Consulting the People of North Manchester', in Huspek, M. (ed.) *Oppositional Discourses and Democracies*. New York: Routledge, pp 40–59. doi: 10.4324/9780203872024.

Basilico, M., Weigel, J., Motgi, A., Bor, J. and Keshavjee S. (2013) 'Health For All?', in Farmer, P., Kim J., Kleinman A., Basilico M. (eds) *Reimagining Global Health: An Introduction*. Berkeley, CA: University of California Press, pp 74–110.

Bassett, L. (2019) 'Corbynism: social democracy in a new left garb', *Political Quarterly*, 90(4): 777–784. doi: 10.1111/1467-923X.12735.

Bassett, L. (2020) *Corbynism and Democracy: A Political Movement In and Against Neoliberalism*. Manchester: University of Manchester.

BBC News (2005) *Target 'putting A&E care at risk'*, *BBC News*. Available at: http://news.bbc.co.uk/1/hi/health/4339653.stm (Accessed: 26 August 2020).

Bear, L. (2014) 'Doubt, conflict, mediation: the anthropology of modern time', *Journal of the Royal Anthropological Institute*, 20(S1): 3–30. doi: 10.1111/1467-9655.12091.

Bear, L. and Mathur, N. (2015) 'Introduction', *The Cambridge Journal of Anthropology*, 33(1): 18–34. doi: 10.3167/ca.2015.330103.

Begley, P. and Sheard, S. (2019) 'McKinsey and the "Tripartite monster": The role of management consultants in the 1974 NHS reorganisation', *Medical History*, 63(4): 390–410. doi: 10.1017/mdh.2019.41.

Berman, Y. and Hovland, T. (2024) *The Impact of Austerity on Mortality and Life Expectancy*. London: LSE International Inequalities Institute. Available at: www.lse.ac.uk/III (Accessed: 26 November 2024).

Bevan, A. (1951) *MR. ANEURIN BEVAN (STATEMENT): HC Deb 23 April 1951 vol 487 cc34-43*, *Hansard*. Available at: https://api.parliament.uk/historic-hansard/commons/1951/apr/23/mr-aneurin-bevan-statement (Accessed: 5 March 2025).

Beyerlein, K. and Bergstrand, K. (2013) 'Biographical availability', in Snow, D. A., della Porta, D., Klandermans, B. and McAdam, D. (eds) *The Wiley-Blackwell Encyclopaedia of Social and Political Movements, Volume 12*. Malden, MA: Wiley Blackwell, pp 137–138.

Bezes, P., Demazière, D., Le Bianic, T., Paradeise, C., Normand, R., Benamouzig, D. et al. (2012) 'New public management and professionals in the public sector. What new patterns beyond opposition?', *Sociologie du Travail*, 54(SUPPL. 1): e1–e52. doi: 10.1016/j.soctra.2012.07.001.

Bhambra, G. (2022) 'Imperial revenue and national welfare: the case of Britain', in Bhambra, G. and McClure, J. (eds) *Imperial Inequalities: The politics of economic governance across European empires*. Manchester: Manchester University Press, pp 198–216.

Bivins, R. (2015) *Contagious Communities: Medicine, Migration, and the NHS in Post War Britain*. Oxford: Oxford University Press.

Blackburn, P. (2018) 'Destination Integration: Big on inspiration, short on legislation - the "quiet revolution" in the NHS', *BMA News*, January 13: 3.

Borsa A., Bejarano, G., Ellen, M. and Bruch, J. (2023) 'Evaluating trends in private equity ownership and impacts on health outcomes, costs, and quality: Systematic review', *BMJ*, 382:e075244. doi: 10.1136/bmj-2023-075244.

Bottery, S. and Jefferies, D. (2025) *Social care 360, The King's Fund*. Available at: https://www.kingsfund.org.uk/insight-and-analysis/long-reads/social-care-360 (Accessed: 5 March 2025).

Boyle, A. and Chiles, T. (2022) *RCEM Acute Insight Series: Beds in the NHS*. London: Royal College of Emergency Medicine. Available at: https://res.cloudinary.com/studio-republic/images/v1653920684/RCEM-Acute-Insight-Series-Beds-1/RCEM-Acute-Insight-Series-Beds-1.pdf?_i=AA (Accessed: 5 March 2023).

Braun, B. and Christophers, B. (2024) 'Asset manager capitalism: an introduction to its political economy and economic geography', *Environment and Planning A*, 56(2): 546–557. doi: 10.1177/0308518X241227743.

Britteon, P., Fatimah, A., Gillibrand, S., Lau, Y., Anselmi, L., Wilson P., et al. (2024) 'The impact of devolution on local health systems: evidence from Greater Manchester, England', *Social Science and Medicine*. Elsevier Ltd, 348(April 2023): 116801. doi: 10.1016/j.socscimed.2024.116801.

Brown, H., Reed, A. and Yarrow, T. (2017) 'Introduction: towards an ethnography of meeting', *Journal of the Royal Anthropological Institute*. doi: 10.1111/1467-9655.12591.

Bruff, I. (2014) 'The rise of authoritarian neoliberalism', *Rethinking Marxism*, 26(1): 113–129. doi: 10.1080/08935696.2013.843250.

Buchan, J. (2023) *Brexit, Covid and the UK's reliance on international recruitment, Nuffield Trust*. Available at: https://www.nuffieldtrust.org.uk/news-item/brexit-covid-and-the-uk-s-reliance-on-international-recruitment (Accessed: 5 March 2025).

Buckingham, H. and Dayan, M. (2019) *Privatisation in the English NHS: fact or fiction?*, *Nuffield Trust*. Available at: https://www.nuffieldtrust.org.uk/news-item/privatisation-in-the-english-nhs-fact-or-fiction (Accessed: 14 August 2020).

Burn-Murdoch, J. (2024) *UK healthcare is already being privatised, but not in the way you think*, *Financial Times*. Available at: https://www.ft.com/content/dbf166ce-1ebb-4a67-980e-9860fd170ba2 (Accessed: 6 March 2025).

Calvert, J. and Arbuthnott, G. (2021) *Failures of State: The Inside Story of Britain's Battle with Coronavirus*. London: Mudlark.

Cameron, S. (2014) David Nicholson – the man who believed in being ruthless with the NHS, *The Telegraph*. Available at: https://www.telegraph.co.uk/news/nhs/10724504/David-Nicholson-the-man-who-believed-in-being-ruthless-with-the-NHS.html (Accessed: 3 February 2017).

Carey, D. (2024) The enormous £90m bill a Greater Manchester hospital is facing: Stepping Hill is facing major issues with its estate, *Manchester Evening News*. Available at: https://www.manchestereveningnews.co.uk/news/greater-manchester-news/enormous-90m-bill-facing-greater-29700980 (Accessed: 6 March 2025).

Carrier, J. G. (2015) 'The concept of class', in Kalb, D. and Carrier, J. G. (eds) *Anthropologies of Class: Power, Practice, and Inequality*. Cambridge: Cambridge University Press, pp 28–40. doi: 10.1017/CBO9781316095867.003.

Carrier, J. G. (2018) 'Moral economy: what's in a name', *Anthropological Theory*, 18(1). doi: 10.1177/1463499617735259.

Charlesworth, A., Watt, T. and Johnson, P. (2018) *Securing the Future: Funding Health and Social Care to the 2030s: Executive Summary*. London: Institute of Fiscal Studies.

Chibber, V. (2022) *The Class Matrix*. Cambridge, MA: Harvard University Press.

Chow, W. S., Ajaz, A. and Priebe, S. (2019) 'What drives changes in institutionalised mental health care? A qualitative study of the perspectives of professional experts', *Social Psychiatry and Psychiatric Epidemiology*, 54(6): 737–744. doi: 10.1007/s00127-018-1634-7.

Christophers, B. (2019) *The New Enclosure: The Appropriation of Public Land in Neoliberal Britain*. London: Verso.

Christophers, B. (2023) *Our Lives in Their Portfolios: Why Asset Managers Own the World*. London: Verso.

Coates, D. and Panitch, L. (2003) 'The continuing relevance of the Milibandian perspective', in Callaghan, J., Fielding, S., and Ludlam, S. (eds) *Interpreting the Labour Party: Approaches to Labour politics and history*. Manchester: Manchester University Press, pp 71–85.

Colbert, M. (2024) How private health has invested in Wes Streeting, *Good Law Project*.

Corporate Watch (2024a) Circle Health & how the world's richest family is honing in on Britain's private hospitals, *Corporate Watch*.

Corporate Watch (2024b) *The National Wealth Service: Privatisation Profiteers*. Available at: https://corporatewatch.org/the-national-wealth-service-privatisation-profiteers/ (Accessed: 12 March 2025).

Cowan, H. (2020) 'Taking the national(ism) out of the national health service: re-locating agency to amongst ourselves', *Critical Public Health*. Taylor & Francis (preprint). doi: 10.1080/09581596.2020.1836328.

Cowan, H. (2024) 'Reframing the public/private debate on healthcare services: tracking boundaries in the National Health Service', *Sociology of Health and Illness*, 46(6): 1152–1168. doi: 10.1111/1467-9566.13758.

Cowan, J. K. (2014) 'Struggling over procedures and other interventions', *HAU: Journal of Ethnographic Theory*, 4(3): 89–97. doi: 10.14318/hau4.3.008.

Cowper, A. (2025) Cowper's Cut 404: 2025's Catch-22 of English health policy and politics – action on fiscal balance, or the RTT backlog?, *Health Policy Insight*.

Crane, J. (2019) '"Save our NHS": activism, information-based expertise and the "new times" of the 1980s', *Contemporary British History*, 33(1): 52–74. doi: 10.1080/13619462.2018.1525299.

Curry, N., Oung, C., Crellin, N. and Dodsworth, E. (2024) *Adult Social Care: What Health and Care Need from the Next Governmen*. London: Nuffield Trust. Available at: https://www.nuffieldtrust.org.uk/resource/what-health-and-care-need-from-the-next-government-2-adult-social-care (Accessed: 12 March 2025).

Cutler, T. (2006) 'A Double Irony? The Politics of National Health Service Expenditure in the 1950s', in Gorsky, M. and Sheard, S. (eds) *Financing Medicine: The British Experience since 1750*. London: Routledge, pp 201–220.

Daniels, S. (2023) *How Consecutive Conservative Governments Destroyed Union Rights – A Timeline of the UK's Anti-strike Laws Since the 1970s*. Lancashire: Edge Hill University.

Dao, A. and Mulligan, J. (2016) 'Toward an anthropology of insurance and health reform: an introduction to the special issue', *Medical Anthropology Quarterly*, 30(1): 5–17.

Darzi, A. (2024) *Independent Investigation of the National Health Service in England*. London: Department of Health and Social Care, gov.uk. Available at: www.nationalarchives.gov.uk/doc/open-government-licence/version/3 (Accessed: 12 March 2025).

Davidson, S. (2021) US company in takeover of network of GP practices, *The Lowdown*. Available at: https://lowdownnhs.info/news/us-takeover-of-a-network-of-gp-practices/ (Accessed: 1 May 2025).

Davis, M. (2003) '"Labourism" and the New Left', in Callaghan, J., Fielding, S., and Ludlam, S. (eds) *Interpreting the Labour Party: Approaches to Labour politics and history*. Manchester: Manchester University Press, pp 39–56.

Day, P. and Klein, R. (1987) *Accountabilities: Five Public Services*. London: Tavistock Publications.

Dayan, M., Gainsbury, S. and Bagri, S. (2024) How has the role of the private sector changed in UK health care?, *Nuffield Trust*. Available at: https://www.nuffieldtrust.org.uk/news-item/how-has-the-role-of-the-private-sector-changed-in-uk-health-care (Accessed: 12 March 2025).

Department of Health (2000) *The NHS Plan: A Plan for Investment. A Plan for Reform*. London: UK Parliament.

Department of Health and Social Care (2025) *Fit for the Future: 10 Year Health Plan*. London: Department of Health and Social Care.

Department of Health and Social Care and Streeting, W. (2025) Faster care for thousands thanks to NHS use of independent sector, *gov.uk*. Available at: https://www.gov.uk/government/news/faster-care-for-thousands-thanks-to-nhs-use-of-independent-sector (Accessed: 13 February 2026).

DHSC Media Team (2024) RAAC in the NHS – media fact sheet, *gov.uk*.

Direct Democracy (2005) Direct Democracy; An Agenda for a New Model Party, *European Business Review*. London: Direct Democracy. doi: 10.1108/ebr.2005.05417eab.006.

Dixon, A., Jones, L. and Mays, N. (2011) *Understanding New Labour's Market Reforms of the English NHS*. London: King's Fund.

Duffy, S. (2014) Personalisation was supposed to empower vulnerable citizens. It failed, *The Guardian*. Available at: https://www.theguardian.com/public-leaders-network/2014/jan/30/personalisation-social-care-support-bureaucracy-service-failure (Accessed: 5 March 2025).

Dulhanty, J. (2022) Greater Manchester won sweeping health powers. But who is holding the system to account?, *The Mill*. Available at: https://manchestermill.co.uk/we-dont-take-scrutiny-seriously-enough/ (Accessed: 3 June 2022).

Dunhill, L. (2018) 'North by North West: where is Greater Manchester's transformation?', *HSJ*. Available at: https://www.hsj.co.uk/finance-and-efficiency/north-by-north-west-where-is-greater-manchesters-transformation/7023180.article (Accessed: 3 June 2022).

Dunhill, L. (2020) 'Greater Manchester must 'deeply recognise' its A&E problem', *HSJ*. Available at: https://www.hsj.co.uk/north-west/greater-manchester-must-deeply-recognise-its-aande-problem/7027025.article (Accessed: 3 June 2022).

Dyer, C. (2022) 'Covid-19: Government's use of VIP lane for awarding PPE contracts was unlawful, says judge', *BMJ*, 376(January): 96. doi: 10.1136/bmj.o96.

Ebbinghaus, B. (2015) 'Welfare Retrenchment', in Wright, J. D. (ed.) *International Encyclopedia of the Social & Behavioral Sciences*. Cambridge: Elsevier Ltd, pp 521–527.

Ehrenreich, B. and Ehrenreich, J. (1977) 'The professional-managerial class', *Radical America*, 11(2): 7–32.

El-Enany, N. (2020) *Bordering Britain: Law, Race and Empire*. Manchester: Manchester University Press.

Eriksen, T. H., Laidlaw, J., Mair, J., Martin, K. and Venkatesan, S. (2015) 'Debate: "the concept of neoliberalism has become an obstacle to the anthropological understanding of the twenty-first century"', *Journal of the Royal Anthropological Institute*, 21(4): 911–923. doi: 10.1111/1467-9655.12294.

Essex, R., Riaz, A., Casalotti, S., Worthing, K., Issa, R., Skinner, J. and Yule A. (2022) 'A decade of the hostile environment and its impact on health', *Journal of the Royal Society of Medicine*, 115(3): 87–90. doi: 10.1177/01410768221078327.

Eurostat (2019) *Health in the European Union – Facts and Figures*. Luxembourg: European Commission.

Evans, D. (2023) *A Nation of Shopkeepers: The Unstoppable Rise of the Petite Bourgeoisie*. London: Repeater.

Evans, G. (2006) *Educational Failure and Working Class White Children in Britain*. London: Palgrave MacMillan.

Evans, G. (2017) 'Brexit Britain: why we are all postindustrial now', *American Ethnologist*, 44(2): 215–219.

Fassin, D. (2012) *Humanitarian Reason: A Moral History of the Present*. Berkeley, CA: University of California Press.

Finn, D. (2019) 'Crosscurrents: Corbyn, Labour and the Brexit crisis', *New Left Review*, 118(July August): 5–35.

Fisher, B. (2024) Nuffield Trust: Funding promised in Budget will meet NHS's day-to-day needs, but won't stretch towards government ambitions to re-build, *Nuffield Trust*. Available at: https://www.nuffieldtrust.org.uk/news-item/funding-promised-in-budget-will-meet-nhs-day-to-day-needs-but-wont-stretch-towards-government-ambitions-to-re-build (Accessed: 6 March 2025).

Fisher, E. and Taylor, B. (2024) NHS hospital care: Who is waiting and what are they waiting for?, *Nuffield Trust*. Available at: https://www.nuffieldtrust.org.uk/news-item/nhs-emergency-and-planned-care-who-is-waiting-and-what-waiting-for (Accessed: 6 March 2024).

Fitzgerald, D., Hinterberger, A., Narayan, J. and Williams, R. (2020) 'Brexit as heredity redux: Imperialism, biomedicine and the NHS in Britain', *Sociological Review*, 68(6): 1161–1178. doi: 10.1177/0038026120914177.

Fong, K. (2024) INQ000474327 – Witness Statement of Dr Kevin Fong, National Clinical Adviser in Emergency Preparedness Resilience and Response (EPRR), dated 06/09/2024, *UK Covid-19 Inquiry*. Available at: https://covid19.public-inquiry.uk/documents/inq000474327-witness-statement-of-dr-kevin-fong-national-clinical-adviser-in-emergency-preparedness-resilience-and-response-eprr-dated-06-09-2024/ (Accessed: 5 March 2025).

Francis, G. (2023) *Free For All: Why the NHS is Worth Saving*. London: Wellcome Collection.

Freedman, S. (2024) *Failed State: Why Nothing Works and How We Fix It*. London: MacMillan.

Gabor, D. (2021) 'The Wall Street consensus', *Development and Change*, 52(3): 429–459. doi: 10.1111/dech.12645.

Garside, J. and Neate, R. (2020) 'UK government "using pandemic to transfer NHS duties to private sector"', *The Guardian*, May. Available at: https://www.theguardian.com/business/2020/may/04/uk-government-using-crisis-to-transfer-nhs-duties-to-private-sector (Accessed: 5 March 2025).

Geertz, C. (1973) 'Thick description: toward an interpretive theory of culture', in Geertz, C. (ed.) *The Interpretation of Culture*. New York: Basic Books, pp 1–17.

General Medical Council (2022) *The state of medical education and practice in the UK*. London: General Medical Council. Available at: http://www.gmc-uk.org/State_of_medicine_Final_web.pdf (Accessed: 5 March 2025).

Gentleman, A. (2019) *The Windrush Betrayal: Exposing the Hostile Environment*. London: Guardian Faber Publishing.

Geoghegan, P. (2024) 'Labour and the lobbyists', *London Review of Books*, 46(16).

Geras, N. (1984) 'The controversy about Marx and justice', *New Left Review*, 33(0): 47–85. doi: 10.21825/philosophica.82563.

Geras, N. (1992) 'Bringing Marx to justice: an addendum and rejoinder', *New Left Review*, 195: 37–69.

Giddens, A. (1994) *Beyond Left and Right: The Future of Radical Politics*. Stanford, CA: Stanford University Press.

Giddens, A. (1998) *The Third Way: The Renewal of Social Democracy*. Cambridge: Polity Press.

Gilburt, H. (2025) NHS reliant on beds in the independent sector for mental health care, *The King's Fund*. Available at: https://www.kingsfund.org.uk/insight-and-analysis/long-reads/nhs-reliant-beds-independent-sector-mental-health-care (Accessed: 13 February 2026).

Gingrich, J. R. (2011) *Making Markets in the Welfare State: The Politics of Varying Market Reforms*. Cambridge: Cambridge University Press.

Ginsburg, F. D. (1989) *Contested Lives: The Abortion Debate in an American Community*. Berkeley, CA: University of California Press.

Gokmenoglu, B. (2022) 'Temporality in the social sciences: new directions for a political sociology of time', *British Journal of Sociology*, 73(3): 643–653. doi: 10.1111/1468-4446.12938.

Goodair, B., Bach-Mortensen, A. M. and Reeves, A. (2024) '"Two sides of the same coin"? A longitudinal analysis evaluating whether financial austerity accelerated NHS privatisation in England 2013–2020', *BMJ Public Health*, 2(1): e000964. doi: 10.1136/bmjph-2024-000964.

Goodair, B. and Reeves, A. (2024) 'The effect of health-care privatisation on the quality of care', *The Lancet Public Health*. The Authors. Published by Elsevier Ltd. This is an Open Access article under the CC BY 4.0 license, 9(3): e199–e206. doi: 10.1016/S2468-2667(24)00003-3.

Gosling, G. (2018) 'Gender, money and professional identity: medical social work and the coming of the British National Health Service', *Women's History Review*, 27(2): 310–328.

Graeber, D. (2001) *Toward an Anthropological Theory of Value: The False Coin of Our Own Dreams*. New York: Palgrave.

Graeber, D. (2013) *The Democracy Project*. London: Penguin Books.

Graeber, D. (2014) 'Anthropology and the rise of the professional-managerial class', *HAU: Journal of Ethnographic Theory*, 4(3): 73–88. doi: 10.14318/hau4.3.007.

Graeber, D. (2020) The Center Blows Itself Up: Care and Spite in the 'Brexit Election', *New York Review of Books*.

Greater Manchester Combined Authority (2015) *Taking Charge of our Health and Social Care in Greater Manchester*. Manchester. Available at: http://www.gmhsc.org.uk/wp-content/uploads/2018/04/GM-Strategic-Plan-Final.pdf%0Ahttp://www.manchester.gov.uk/info/100004/the_council_and_democracy/66/councils_in_greater_manchester/1%0Ahttp://www.manchester.gov.uk/info/100004/the_council_and_democracy/66 (Accessed: 5 March 2025).

Greenhalgh, T. and McKee, M. (2025) 'Physician associates and anaesthetic associates in UK: rapid systematic review of recent UK based research', *BMJ*, (388): e084613. doi: 10.1136/bmj-2025-084613.

Greer, I. and Umney, C. (2022) *Marketization: How Capitalist Exchange Disciplines and Subverts Democracy*. London: Bloomsbury Academic.

Griffiths, T. (1997) *Food for Ravens*. London: Oberon Books.

Groce, N. and Groce, N. E. (2020) 'In the US, even those with excellent healthcare insurance plans struggle', *BMJ*, 368: m808.

Guyer, J. (1995) *Money Matters: Instability, Values and Social Payments in the Modern History of West African Communities*. Melton: James Currey.

Haider, A. (2016) Bernstein in Seattle: Representative Democracy and the Revolutionary Subject (Part 1), *Viewpoint Magazine*.

Ham, C. (2018) Making sense of integrated care systems, integrated care partnerships and accountable care organisations in the NHS in England, *The King's Fund*. Available at: https://www.kingsfund.org.uk/publications/making-sense-integrated-care-systems#acos (Accessed: 21 August 2020).

Ham, C. (2023) *The rise and decline of the NHS in England 2000–20*. London: King's Fund. Available at: https://assets.kingsfund.org.uk/f/256914/x/0ab966500b/rise_decline_nhs_england_2000-20_2023.pdf (Accessed: 5 March 2025).

Hammond, J., Speed E., Allen P., McDermott I., Coleman A., Checkland K. (2018) 'Autonomy, accountability, and ambiguity in arm's-length meta-governance: the case of NHS England', *Public Management Review*, 21(8): 1148–1169. doi: 10.1080/14719037.2018.1544660.

Hancock, M. (2019) Tweet, *Twitter*. Available at: https://twitter.com/MattHancock/status/1195997609942560768 (Accessed: 5 March 2021).

Hannah, S. (2018) *The Labour Left: A Party with Socialists in It*. London: Pluto Press.

Hayes, L. (2017) *Stories of Care: A Labour of Law*. London: Palgrave MacMillan.

Health and Social Care Committee (2018) Integrated care: organisations, partnerships and systems: seventh report of session 2017–19: report, together with formal minutes relating to the report, *House of Commons papers. Session 2017–19;* London. Available at: https://www.parliament.uk/business/committees/committees-a-z/commons-select/health-committee/inquiries/parliament-2017/inquiry4/%0Ahttps://www.parliament.uk/documents/commons-committees/Health/Correspondence/2017-19/Government-response-to-Committee-report (Accessed: 5 March 2021).

Hewison, A. (2002) 'Managerial values and rationality in the UK national health service', *Public Management Review*, 4(4): 549–580. doi: 10.1080/14616670210164762.

Hiam, L., Dorling, D., Harrison, D. and McKee, M. (2017) 'What caused the spike in mortality in England and Wales in January 2015?', *Journal of the Royal Society of Medicine*, 110(4): 131–137. doi: 10.1177/0141076817693600.

Hood, C. (2010) *The Blame Game: Spin, Bureaucracy, and Self-Preservation in Government*. Princeton, NJ: Princeton University Press.

Hood, C. and Dixon, R. (2015) 'What we have to show for 30 years of new public management: higher costs, more complaints', *Governance*, 28(3): 265–267. doi: 10.1111/gove.12150.

Horton, S., Abadía, C., Mulligan, J. and Thompson, J. (2014) 'Critical anthropology of global health "takes a stand" statement: a critical medical anthropological approach to the U.S.'s affordable care act', *Medical Anthropology Quarterly*, 28(1): 1–22.

Hughes, L. (2024) Demand for private healthcare hits record high in UK, *Financial Times*. Available at: https://www.ft.com/content/a4f07a08-b7e9-4330-9915-c2640edf7866?segmentId=bf7fa2fd-67ee-cdfa-8261-b2a3edbdf916 (Accessed: 6 March 2025).

Hughes, L. and Borrett, A. (2024) Why does the NHS have a productivity problem?, *Financial Times*. Available at: https://www.ft.com/content/0dc04f38-249e-4ae0-af96-62e35e813259 (Accessed: 6 March 2025).

Hughes, L. and Borrett, A. (2025) 'Evolution not revolution': Can the private sector help cut NHS waiting lists?, *The Financial Times*. Available at: https://www.ft.com/content/2c50e709-7baa-49d9-8d19-6cdc22507e46?desktop=true&segmentId=d8d3e364-5197-20eb-17cf-2437841d178a#myft:notification:instant-email:content (Accessed: 12 March 2025).

Hunter, B. M. (2025) 'Internationalisation and moral economies in healthcare: NHS exporting and the English patient', *Globalization and Health. BioMed Central*, 21(37): 1–13. doi: 10.1186/s12992-025-01122-7.

Hyde, M. (2022) What's more cringey than a Matt Hancock bushtucker trial? The Tory MPs voting for it, *The Guardian*. Available at: https://www.theguardian.com/commentisfree/2022/nov/11/cringey-matt-hancock-bushtucker-trial-im-a-celebrity (Accessed: 5 March 2025).

Hyman, R. and Brough, I. (1975) *Social Values and Industrial Relations: A Study of Fairness and Equality*. Oxford: Basic Blackwell.

Iacobucci, G. (2014) 'Senior Tories admit NHS reorganisation was worst mistake since being in government', *BMJ*, 349(October): g6221. doi: 10.1136/bmj.g6221.

Independent Healthcare Providers Network (2025) *IHPN Quarterly Data – NHS Activity, January 2025*. Available at: https://www.ihpn.org.uk/ihpn-quarterly-nhs-stats-january-2025/ (Accessed: 12 March 2025).

Investegate (2019) Spire Healthcare reports its results for the year ended 31 December 2018, *RNS, London Stock Exchange*.

Irons, R. (2024) 'Diversity amongst decision makers? Workplace inequality, black underrepresentation, and the afterlife of colonialism in NHS governance', *Medicine Anthropology Theory*, 11(2): 1–22. doi: 10.17157/mat.11.2.7305.

Jefferies, D., Wellings, D., Morris, J. and Lobont, C. (2024) *Public Satisfaction with the NHS and Social Care in 2023: Results from the British Social Attitudes Survey*. London: The King's Fund.

Jenkins, S. (2015) The secret negotiations to restore Manchester to greatness, *The Guardian*. Available at: https://www.theguardian.com/uk-news/2015/feb/12/secret-negotiations-restore-manchester-greatness (Accessed: 14 August 2020).

Jones, L. (2016) *Policy as Discursive Practice: An Ethnographic Study of Hospital Planning in England*. London School of Hygiene & Tropical Medicine. doi: 10.17037/PUBS.02997234.

Jones, L. and Armit, K. (2025) 'Doctors as system leaders: medical professionalism and "making a stand"', *Social Science and Medicine*, 381(October 2024): 118314. doi: 10.1016/j.socscimed.2025.118314.

Jones, L. and Exworthy, M. (2015) 'Framing in policy processes: a case study from hospital planning in the National Health Service in England', *Social Science & Medicine*, 124: 196–204.

Kang, C., Tomkow, L. and Farrington, R. (2019) 'Access to primary health care for asylum seekers and refugees: a qualitative study of service user experiences in the UK', *British Journal of General Practice*, 69(685): e537–e545. doi: 10.3399/bjgp19x701309.

Kapadia, D., Zhang, J., Salway, S., Nazroo, J., Booth, A., Villarroel-Williams, N., Bécares, L. and Esmai, L. (2022) *Ethnic Inequalities in Healthcare: A Rapid Evidence Review – NHS – Race and Health ObservatoryNHS – Race and Health Observatory*. London: NHS Race and Health Observatory. Available at: https://www.nhsrho.org/publications/ethnic-inequalities-in-healthcare-a-rapid-evidence-review/ (Accessed: 12 March 2025).

Kapferer, B. and Gold, M. (eds) (2018) *Moral Anthropology: A Critique*. New York: Berghahn Books.

Keane, W. (2007) *Christian Moderns: Freedom and Fetish in the Mission Encounter*. Berkeley, CA: University of California Press.

Keane, W. (2010) 'Minds, Surfaces, and Reasons in the Anthropology of Ethics', in Lambek, M. (ed.) *Ordinary Ethics: Anthropology, Language, and Action*. New York: Fordham University Press, pp 64–83.

Keeble, E., Bardsley, M., Durand, M., Hoomans, T. and Mays, N. (2019) 'Area level impacts on emergency hospital admissions of the integrated care and support pioneer programme in England: difference-in-differences analysis', *BMJ Open*, 9(8): 1–7. doi: 10.1136/bmjopen-2018-026509.

Kerslake, B. (2017) I'm quitting as a hospital boss: dire NHS funding problems give me no choice, *The Guardian*. Available at: https://www.theguardian.com/commentisfree/2017/dec/10/quit-hospital-boss-nhs-chair-kings-college-hospital-london (Accessed: 12 March 2020).

Kirkup, J. and Winnett, R. (2012) Theresa May interview: 'We're going to give illegal migrants a really hostile reception', *The Telegraph*, 25 May. Available at: https://www.telegraph.co.uk/news/uknews/immigration/9291483/Theresa-May-interview-Were-going-to-give-illegal-migrants-a-really-hostile-reception.html (Accessed: 12 March 2020).

Kirkwood, G., Pollock, A. M. and Roderick, P. (2024) 'Private sector expansion and the widening NHS treatment gap between rich and poor in England: Admissions for NHS-funded elective primary hip and knee replacements between 1997/98 and 2018/19', *Health Policy*, 146(June): 105118. doi: 10.1016/j.healthpol.2024.105118.

Koch, I. (2017) 'Brexit beyond culture wars', *American Ethnologist*, 44(2): 225–230.

Koch, I. (2018) *Personalizing the State: An Anthropology of Law, Politics, and Welfare in Austerity Britain*. Oxford: Oxford University Press.

Koram, K. (2022) *Uncommon Wealth: Britain and the Aftermath of Empire*. London: John Murray.

Krachler, N. (2013) *How to Create the Conditions for a Healthcare Market: The Step-by-step Marketisation of the NHS in England – An Outline of Marketisation Processes in the English NHS On The Basis of Marketization Theory*. London: University of Greenwich.

Krachler, N. and Greer, I. (2015) 'When does marketisation lead to privatisation? Profit-making in English health services after the 2012 Health and Social Care Act', *Social Science and Medicine*, 124: 215–223. doi: 10.1016/j.socscimed.2014.11.045.

Laidlaw, J. (2014) *The Subject of Virtue: An Anthropology of Ethics and Freedom*. Cambridge: Cambridge University Press.

Laidlaw, J. (2023) 'Introduction', in Laidlaw, J. (ed.) *The Cambridge Handbook for the Anthropology of Ethics*. Cambridge: Cambridge University Press, pp 1–32.

LaingBuisson (2025) Independent sector mental health hospitals market valued at record £2.36 billion, as occupancy rates in NHS mental health units reach highest recorded levels, *LaingBuisson Intelligence + Insight* Available at: https://www.laingbuisson.com/press-releases/independent-sector-mental-health-hospitals-market-valued-at-record-2-36-billion/ (Accessed: 12 March 2025).

Lazar, S. (2023) 'Activism and Political Organization', in Laidlaw, J. (ed.) *The Cambridge Handbook for the Anthropology of Ethics*. Cambridge: Cambridge University Press, pp 791–816. doi: 10.1017/9781108591249.031.

Lethbridge, J. (2012) *Empty Promises: The Impact of Outsourcing on NHS Services*. London: Unison.

Levi, M. and Olsen, D. (2000) 'The Battles in Seattle', *Politics and Society*, 28(3): 309–329.

Lewis, J. and Glennerster, H. (1996) *Implementing the New Community Care*. Buckingham: Open University Press.

Leys, C. (2016) 'The English NHS: from market failure to trust, professionalism and democracy', *Soundings*, 64: 11–40.

Leys, C. and Player, S. (2011) *The Plot Against the NHS*. Pontypool, UK: Merlin Press.

Little, G. and Sharp, E. (2023) *Lessons in Organising: What Trade Unionists Can Learn from the War on Teachers*. London: Pluto Press.

Lonergan, G. (2020) 'Who is a "temporary migrant"? Deservingness, Nationalism and Migrant Access to the NHS', in Follis, L., Burns, N. and Follis, K. (eds) *Healthcare Mobilities and National Health Systems*. Lancaster: Lancaster University, pp 9–14.

Lonergan, G. (2023) 'Reproduction and the expanding border: pregnant migrants as a "problem" in the 2014 Immigration Act', *Sociology*, OnlineFirs. doi: 10.1177/00380385231157987.

Lorne, C. and Lambert, M. (2023) '"Protecting the NHS" – and its limits', *Soundings*, 82(82): 61–74. doi: 10.3898/soun.82.04.2022.

Mallorie, S. (2024) NHS workforce in a nutshell, *The King's Fund*. Available at: https://www.kingsfund.org.uk/insight-and-analysis/data-and-charts/nhs-workforce-nutshell (Accessed: 5 March 2025).

Manchester University Foundation Trust (2024) *Manchester University NHS Foundation Trust Annual Report and Accounts 1st April 2022 to 31st March 2023*. Manchester: Manchester University Foundation Trust. Available at: https://mft.nhs.uk/the-trust/reports-and-publications/ (Accessed: 5 March 2025).

Marmot, M., Allen, J., Goldblatt, P., Herd, E. and Morrison, J. (2020) *Build Back Fairer: The Covid-19 Marmot Review*. London. Available at: https://www.health.org.uk/publications/build-back-fairer-the-covid-19-marmot-review (Accessed: 5 March 2025).

Marmot, M., Allen, J., Boyce, T., Goldblatt, P. and Morrison, J. (2020) *Health Equity in England: The Marmot Review 10 Years On*. London: The Institute of Health Equity.

Marsh, S. and Garcia, C. A. (2024) Private equity groups collecting millions to run UK government-funded sexual assault referral centres, *The Guardian*. Available at: https://www.theguardian.com/business/2024/mar/13/uk-private-equity-firms-sexual-assault-referral-centres (Accessed: 5 March 2025).

Mattingly, C. (2014a) 'Moral deliberation and the agentive self in Laidlaw's ethics', *HAU: Journal of Ethnographic Theory*, 4(1): 473–486. doi: 10.14318/hau4.1.030.

Mattingly, C. (2014b) *Moral Laboratories: Family Peril and the Struggle for a Good Life*. Oakland, CA: University of California Press.

Mazzucato, M. and Collington, R. (2023) *The Big Con: How the Consulting Industry Weakens our Businesses, Infantilizes our Governments and Warps our Economies*. London: Allen Lane.

McCarthy, M. A. and Desan, M. H. (2023) 'The problem of class abstractionism', *Sociological Theory*, 41(1): 3–26. doi: 10.1177/07352751231152489.

McLellan, A. (2024) 'The return of austerity to the NHS means making tough choices', *Health Service Journal*. Available at: https://www.hsj.co.uk/policy-and-regulation/the-return-of-austerity-to-the-nhs-means-making-tough-choices/7038276.article?ref=healthpolicyinsight.com (Accessed: 12 March 2025).

Merry, L. and Gainsbury, S. (2023) What was austerity's toll on the NHS before the pandemic?, *Nuffield Trust*. Available at: https://www.nuffieldtrust.org.uk/news-item/what-was-austeritys-toll-on-the-nhs-before-the-pandemic (Accessed: 5 March 2025).

Miliband, R. (2009) *Parliamentary Socialism: A Study in the Politics of Labour*. London: Merlin Press.

Millard, C. (2020) 'Using personal experience in the academic medical humanities: a genealogy', *Social Theory and Health*, 18(2): 184–198. doi: 10.1057/s41285-019-00089-x.

Moskalenko, E. (2020) Student loans in the public sector finances: a methodological guide, *Office for National Statistics*. Available at: https://www.ons.gov.uk/economy/governmentpublicsectorandtaxes/publicsectorfinance/methodologies/studentloansinthepublicsectorfinancesamethodologicalguide/pdf (Accessed: 8 March 2025).

Mosse, D., Baker, D., Carroll, M., Chase, L., Kloocke, R., Wickremasinghe, K., et al. (2023) 'The contribution of anthropology to the study of Open Dialogue: ethnographic research methods and opportunities', *Frontiers in Psychology*, 14(May): 1–14. doi: 10.3389/fpsyg.2023.1111588.

Muehlebach, A. (2012) *The Moral Neoliberal: Welfare and Citizenship in Italy*. Chicago, IL: University of Chicago Press.

Munn, N. D. (1986) *The Fame of Gawa: A Symbolic Study of Value Transformation in a Massim (Papua New Guinea) Society*. Cambridge: Cambridge University Press.

Nairn, T. (1964a) 'The Nature of the Labour Party (Part I)', *New Left Review*, (27).

Nairn, T. (1964b) 'The Nature of the Labour Party (Part II)', *New Left Review*, (28).

Narotzky, S. (2016) 'Between inequality and injustice: dignity as a motive for mobilization during the crisis', *History and Anthropology*, 27(1): 74–92. doi: 10.1080/02757206.2015.1111209.

Narotzky, S. (2019) 'Response to Webb Keane: how everyday ethics becomes a moral economy, and vice versa', *Economics: The Open-Access, Open-Assessment E-Journal*, 13(46). Available at: http://www.economics-ejournal.org/economics/discussionpapers/2019-9/comment.2019-04-04.5579831842/at_download/file (Accessed: 4 March 2021).

National Audit Office (2019) *NHS financial sustainability: Key facts*. London, UK. Available at: https://www.nao.org.uk/wp-content/uploads/2019/01/NHS-financial-sustainability_.pdf (Accessed: 5 August 2020).

National Audit Office (2020a) *Investigation into the rescue of Carillion's PFI hospital contracts*. Available at: https://www.nao.org.uk/reports/investigation-into-the-rescue-of-carillions-pfi-hospital-contracts/?nab=1 (Accessed: 5 March 2025).

National Audit Office (2020b) *The government's approach to test and trace in England: interim report*. Available at: https://www.nao.org.uk/reports/the-governments-approach-to-test-and-trace-in-england-interim-report/ (Accessed: 5 March 2025).

National Audit Office (2021) *Test and Trace in England progress update*. London. Available at: https://www.nao.org.uk/wp-content/uploads/2021/06/Test-and-trace-in-England-progress-update.pdf (Accessed: 5 March 2025).

Nazroo, J. and Bécares, L. (2021) *Ethnic inequalities in COVID-19 mortality: A consequence of persistent racism, Runnymede/CoDE Covid Briefings*. London: Runnymede Trust. Available at: https://www.runnymedetrust.org/publications/ethnic-inequalities-in-covid-19-mortality-a-consequence-of-persistent-racism (Accessed: 5 March 2025).

Neville, S. (2025) Ex-NHS boss Amanda Pritchard: 'You can't change your mind every five minutes', *The Financial Times*. Available at: https://www.ft.com/content/5cf4de5b-604f-4247-adc3-a473dc241cc9 (Accessed: 1 May 2025).

Newman, M. (2003) 'Ralph Miliband and the Labour Party: from Parliamentary Socialism to "Bennism"', in Callaghan, J., Fielding, S., and Ludlam, S. (eds) *Interpreting the Labour Party: Approaches to Labour politics and History*. Manchester: Manchester University Press, pp 57–70.

NHS Confederation (2022) *System on a cliff edge: addressing challenges in social care capacity*. Available at: https://www.nhsconfed.org/publications/system-cliff-edge-addressing-challenges-social-care-capacity (Accessed: 5 March 2025).

NHS Employers (2025) *The history of pay in the NHS, NHS Employers*. Available at: https://www.nhsemployers.org/articles/history-pay-nhs (Accessed: 1 May 2025).

NHS England (2014) *5 Year Forward View*. Available at: https://www.england.nhs.uk/publication/nhs-five-year-forward-view/ (Accessed: 5 March 2020).

NHS England (2024a) *Consultant-led Referral to Treatment Waiting Times Data 2024–25, NHS England*. Available at: https://www.england.nhs.uk/statistics/statistical-work-areas/rtt-waiting-times/rtt-data-2024-25/#Dec24 (Accessed: 6 March 2025).

NHS England (2024b) *Independent Review of Greater Manchester Mental Health NHS Foundation Trust*. London: NHS England.

O'Grady, T. (2022) *The Transformation of British Welfare Policy: Politics, Discourse, and Public Opinion*. Oxford: Oxford University Press.

O'Toole, G. (2023) Required reading for the Labour party, *Morning Star*. Available at: https://morningstaronline.co.uk/article/c/required-reading-labour-party (Accessed: 26 August 2025).

Office for National Statistics (2020) *Deaths involving COVID-19 by local area and socioeconomic deprivation: deaths occurring between 1 March and 30 June 2020*. Available at: https://www.ons.gov.uk/peoplepopulationandcommunity/birthsdeathsandmarriages/deaths/datasets/deathsinvolvingcovid19bylocalareaanddeprivation (Accessed: 3 March 2025).

Oliver, D. (2014) 'Stop wasting taxpayers' money on management consultancy for the NHS', *BMJ*, 349: g7243. doi: 10.1136/bmj.g7243.

Ormerod, J. (2018a) Legislation, Privatisation and the NHS, *Socialist Health Association*. Available at: https://www.sochealth.co.uk/2018/06/13/34928/ (Accessed: 13 August 2020).

Ormerod, J. (2018b) Privatisation from the top-down: the corporate sector and decision-making, *Socialist Health Association*. Available at: https://sochealth.co.uk/2018/06/08/privatisation-from-the-top-down-the-corporate-sector-and-decision-making/ (Accessed: 13 August 2020).

Ormerod, J. (2018c) The great NHS property sell-off gathers pace, *openDemocracy*. Available at: https://www.opendemocracy.net/en/great-nhs-property-sell-off-gathers-pace/ (Accessed: 13 August 2020).

Ortner, S. B. (2016) 'Dark anthropology and its others Theory since the eighties', *Journal of Ethnographic Theory*, 6(1): 47–73.

Palomera, J. and Vetta, T. (2016) 'Moral economy: Rethinking a radical concept', *Anthropological Theory*, 16(4): 1–21.

Park, A., Curtice, J., Clery, E. and Bryson, C. (2012) *British Social Attitudes: The 27th Report: Exploring Labour's Legacy*. London: Sage Publications Ltd.

Parry, J. (2020) *Classes of Labour: Work and Life in a Central Indian Steel Town*. London: Routledge.

Pedersen, S. (2018) 'One-man ministry', *London Review of Books2*, 40(3).

Penna, D. (2024) Streeting hits out at 'middle-class Lefties' opposed to Labour NHS plans, *The Telegraph*. Available at: https://www.telegraph.co.uk/politics/2024/04/08/streeting-middle-class-lefties-opposed-to-labour-nhs-plans/ (Accessed: 12 March 2025).

Polanyi, K. (2001) *The Great Transformation: The Political and Economic Origins of Our Time*. Boston, MA: Beacon Press.

Pollock, A. M. (2020) Thanks to outsourcing, England's test and trace system is in chaos, *The Guardian*, July. Available at: https://www.theguardian.com/commentisfree/2020/jul/31/outsourcing-england-test-trace-nhs-private (Accessed: 12 March 2025).

Potter, J. L. (2015) 'Providing accessible healthcare to migrants is morally right and cost effective', *BMJ*, 351: h3775. doi: 10.1136/bmj.h3775.

Potter, J. L., Burman, M., Tweed, C., Vanghuela, D., White, V., Swinglehurst, D., et al. (2017) 'S27 Have recent changes to health policies increased diagnostic delay amongst migrant patients with active TB?', *Thorax*, 72: A20. doi: 10.1136/thoraxjnl-2017-210983.33.

Povinelli, E. A. (2011) *Economies of Abandonment: Social Belonging and Endurance in Late Liberalism*. Durham, NC: Duke University Press.

Power, M. (1999) *The Audit Society: Rituals of Verification*. Oxford: Oxford University Press.

Power, M. (2000) 'The audit society – second thoughts', *International Journal of Auditing*, 4(1): 111–119. doi: 10.1111/1099-1123.00306.

Power, S. (2018) 'Remembering and Imagining in Human Development: Fairness and Social Movements in Ireland', in Saint-Laurent, C. de, Obradović, S., and Kevin R. Carriere (eds) *Imagining Collective Futures: Perspectives from Social, Cultural and Political Psychology*. London: Palgrave MacMillan, pp 221–236.

Press, A. and Ehrenreich, B. (2019) *On the Origins of the Professional-Managerial Class: An Interview with Barbara Ehrenreich*, Dissent. Available at: https://dissentmagazine.org/online_articles/on-the-origins-of-the-professional-managerial-class-an-interview-with-barbara-ehrenreich/ (Accessed: 20 August 2020).

Prime Minister's Office (2020) *Prime Minister's statement on coronavirus (COVID-19): 31 October 2020*, gov.uk. Available at: https://www.gov.uk/government/speeches/prime-ministers-statement-on-coronavirus-covid-19-31-october-2020 (Accessed: 12 January 2021).

Prime Minister's Office (2021) *Prime Minister's address to the nation: 4 January 2021*, gov.uk. Available at: https://www.gov.uk/government/speeches/prime-ministers-address-to-the-nation-4-january-2021 (Accessed: 12 January 2021).

Prince, R. J. (2014) 'Situating Health and the Public in Africa: Historical and Anthropological Perspectives', in Prince, R. J. and Marsland, R. (eds) *Making and Unmaking Public Health in Africa: Ethnographic and Historical Perspectives*. Athens: Ohio University Press, pp 1–53.

Public Accounts Committee (2015) *Circle's withdrawal from Hinchingbrooke Hospital update report published*, UK Parliament. Available at: https://committees.parliament.uk/committee/127/public-accounts-committee/news/185264/report-circle-withdrawal-from-hinchingbrooke-hospital/ (Accessed: 5 March 2025).

Pushkar, P. (2012) NHS: Competition and Privatisation, *Now Then Magazine*. Available at: http://nowthenmagazine.com/sheffield/issue-45/nhs/ (Accessed: 3 February 2016).

Pushkar, P. (2017) I'm A Doctor – Not A Proxy Border Guard, *Huffington Post*.

Pushkar, P. (2019) 'NHS Activism: The Limits and Potentialities of a New Solidarity', *Medical Anthropology*, 38(3): 239–252. doi: 10.1080/01459740.2018.1532421.

Pushkar, P. (2023) 'Accountabilities in the NHS: Coercion, Finance and Responsibility', *The Cambridge Journal of Anthropology*, 41(1): 118–136. doi: 10.3167/cja.2023.410109.

Pushkar, P. (2024) 'Ethnographers and Subjectivity; Doctors and Comradely Critique', in Greco, C. (ed.) *Politics and Practices of the Ethnographies of Biomedicine and STEM: Among White Coats*. Cham: Palgrave MacMillan, pp 45–63. doi: 10.1007/978-3-031-65797-9.

Pushkar, P. and Tomkow, L. (2021) 'Clinician-led evidence-based activism: a critical analysis', *Critical Public Health*, 31(2): 235–244. doi: 10.1080/09581596.2020.1841112.

Pushkar, P. and Tomkow, L. (2025) 'The universalising medium has stopped universalising: The vertical and horizontal retrenchment of citizenship in austerity Britain', in Follis, F., Burns, N. and Follis, K. (eds) *Migrant and refugee access to health systems: Challenging (im)mobilities in healthcare*. Cheltenham: Edward Elgar Publishing, pp 183–196.

Reed, J. (2024) *How close were hospitals to collapse in Covid?*, BBC. Available at: https://www.bbc.co.uk/news/articles/c78dl0xv7y2o (Accessed: 5 March 2025).

Reed, S., Schlepper, L. and Edwards, N. (2022) *Health system recovery from Covid-19: International lessons for the NHS*, Nuffield Trust. Available at: https://www.nuffieldtrust.org.uk/research/health-system-recovery-from-covid-19-international-lessons-for-the-nhs#key-findings- (Accessed: 5 March 2025).

Robbins, J. (2013) 'Beyond the suffering subject: toward an anthropology of the good', *Journal of the Royal Anthropological Institute*, 19(3): 447–462.

Robbins, J. (2015) 'Ritual, value, and example: on the perfection of cultural representations', *Journal of the Royal Anthropological Institute*, 21(S1): 18–29. doi: 10.1111/1467-9655.12163.

Robinson, E. (2017) 'Recapturing Our Traditions? The Rhetorical Shift from New to One Nation Labour (and Beyond)', in Atkins, J. and Gaffney, J. (eds) *Voices of the UK Left. Rhetoric, Politics and Society*. Cham: Palgrave MacMillan, pp 39–59.

Rodriguez Santana, I., Aragón, M., Rice, N. and Mason, A. (2020) 'Trends in and drivers of healthcare expenditure in the English NHS: a retrospective analysis', *Health Economics Review*, 10(1): 1–11. doi: 10.1186/s13561-020-00278-9.

Rose, N. (1992) 'Governing the enterprising self', in Heelas, P. and Morris, P. (eds) *The Values of the Enterprise Culture: The Moral Debate*. London: Routledge, pp 141–164.

Rose, N. (2000) 'Community, citizenship and the third way', *American Behavioral Scientist*, 43(9): 1395–1411.

Rosen, R. (2025) *A short history of the GP contract and its evolution in England*, Nuffield Trust. Available at: https://www.nuffieldtrust.org.uk/news-item/a-short-history-of-the-gp-contract-and-its-evolution-in-england (Accessed: 12 March 2025).

Rossen, B. and Faroque, A. (2016) 'Diagnosing the causes of rising health-care expenditure in Canada: does Baumol's cost disease loom large?', *American Journal of Health Economics*, 2(2): 184–212. doi: 10.1162/ajhe_a_00041.

Rowland, D. (2019) *Flawed data? Why NHS spending on the independent sector may actually be much more than 7%*, LSE Blogs. Available at: https://blogs.lse.ac.uk/politicsandpolicy/nhs-spending-on-the-independent-sector/ (Accessed: 12 March 2025).

Rowland, D. (2022) *Briefing note: the bet against the NHS – how likely is a two-tier healthcare system in the UK?* London: Centre for Health and the Public Interest.

Rowland, D. (2025) *Out of Sight – the hidden profits and conflicts of interest behind the outsourcing of NHS cataract care*, CHPI. Available at: https://www.chpi.org.uk/reports/out-of-sight-the-hidden-profits-and-conflicts-of-interest-at-behind-the-outsourcing-of-nhs-cataract-care (Accessed: 1 May 2025).

Royal College of Emergency Medicine (2017) *Written evidence submitted on behalf of the Royal College of Emergency Medicine, UK Government Health Select Committee*. Available at: http://data.parliament.uk/writtenevidence/committeeevidence.svc/evidencedocument/health-committee/sustainability-and-transformation-partnerships/written/76851.html (Accessed: 20 September 2019).

Royal College of Nursing (2025) *On the frontline of the UK's corridor care crisis*. London: Royal College of Nursing.

Saunders, J. (2016) *Working for the NHS, People's History of the NHS*. Available at: https://peopleshistorynhs.org/working-for-the-nhs/ (Accessed: 12 March 2025).

Saunders, J. (2022) 'The making of "NHS staff" as a worker identity, 1948–85', in Crane, J. and Hand, J. (eds) *Posters, protests, and prescriptions: Cultural Histories of the NHS*. Manchester: Manchester University Press, pp 25–53.

Scally, G., Jacobson, B. and Abbasi, K. (2020) 'The UK's public health response to covid-19', *BMJ*, 369: m1932. doi: 10.1136/bmj.m1932.

Schmidt, I. (2015) 'Farewell to Europe's Working Classes: Welcome the Making of the European Working Class?', in Bieler, A., Erne, R., Golden, D., Helle, I., Kjeldstadli, K., Matos, T. and Stan, S. (eds) *Labour and Transnational Action in Times of Crisis*. London: Rowman & Littlefield International, Ltd., pp 29–40.

Scobie, S. (2019) *Are patients benefitting from better integrated care?', QualityWatch blog.*, Nuffield Trust. Available at: https://www.nuffieldtrust.org.uk/news-item/are-patients-benefiting-from-better-integrated-care (Accessed: 28 February 2020).

Scott, J. (1991) 'The evidence of experience', *Critical Enquiry*, 17(4): 773–797.

Seaton, A. (2023) *Our NHS: A History of Britain's Best-Loved Institution*. New Haven, CT: Yale University Press.

Shore, C. and Wright, S. (1997) 'Policy: A new field of anthropology', in Shore, C. and Wright, S. (eds) *Anthropology of Policy: Perspectives on Governance and Power*. Abingdon: Routledge, pp 3–39.

Shore, C. and Wright, S. (2011) 'Conceptualising Policy: Technologies of governance and the politics of visibility', in Shore, C., Wright, S., and Però, D. (eds) *Policy Worlds*. Oxford: Berghahn Books, pp 1–25.

Shore, C. and Wright, S. (2015) 'Audit culture revisited: rankings, ratings, and the reassembling of society', *Current Anthropology*, 56(3): 421–444. doi: 10.1086/681534.

Silver, B. J. (2003) *Forces of Labour: Workers' Movements and Globalization Since 1870*. Cambridge: Cambridge University Press.

Simpson, J. M. (2018) *Migrant Architects of the NHS: South Asian Doctors and the Reinvention of British General Practice (1940s–1980s)*. Manchester: Manchester University Press.

Skeggs, B. (1997) *Formations of Class and Gender: Becoming Respectable*. London: Sage Publications Ltd.

Skeggs, B. and Loveday, V. (2012) 'Struggles for value: value practices, injustice, judgment, affect and the idea of class', *British Journal of Sociology*, 63(3): 472–490. doi: 10.1111/j.1468-4446.2012.01420.x.

Slobodian, Q. (2018) *Globalists: The End of Empire and the Birth of Neoliberalism*. Cambridge, MA: Harvard University Press.

Slothuus, L. (2021) 'Comradely Critique', *Political Studies*, online fir: 1–19. doi: 10.1177/00323217211040011.

Smith, K. (2012) 'Anxieties of Englishness and participation in democracy', *Focaal*, (62): 30–41.

Smith, K. and Staples, J. (2015) 'Introduction: The Interview as Analytical Category', in Smith, K., Staples, J., and Rapport, N. (eds) *Extraordinary Encounters: Authenticity and the Interview*. New York: Berghahn Books, pp 1–18.

Sotirakopoulos, N. and Rootes, C. (2014) 'Occupy London in International and Local Context', in Porta, D. Della and Mattoni, A. (eds) *Spreading Protest: Social Movements in Times of Crisis*. Colchester: ECPR Press, pp 171–191.

Stanley, L. (2022) *Britain Alone: How a Decade of Conflict Remade the Nation*. Manchester: Manchester University Press.

Stedman-Jones, G. (1983) *Languages of Class: Studies in English Working Class History*. Cambridge: Cambridge University Press.

Stewart, E. et al. (2022) 'Doing "our bit": Solidarity, inequality, and COVID-19 crowdfunding for the UK National Health Service', *Social Science and Medicine*, 308(March). doi: 10.1016/j.socscimed.2022.115214.

Stewart, J. (1999) *The Battle for Health: A Political History of the Socialist Medical Association, 1930–51*. London: Routledge Revivals.

Strathern, M. (1997) 'From improvement to enhancement: An anthropological comment on the audit culture', *The Cambridge Journal of Anthropology*, 19(3): 1–21.

Strathern, M. (2000a) *Audit Cultures: Anthropological Studies in Accountability, Ethics and the Academy*. London: Routledge. doi: 10.1038/378457a0.

Strathern, M. (2000b) 'Introduction: New Accountabilities', in Strathern, M. (ed.) *Audit Cultures: Anthropological Studies in Accountability, Ethics and the Academy*. London: Routledge, pp 1–18.

Student Loans Company (no date) *Our governance*, gov.uk. Available at: https://www.gov.uk/government/organisations/student-loans-company/about/our-governance (Accessed: 12 March 2025).

Talora, J. (2024) Private provider takes over NHS services worth £1.3bn, *Health Service Journal.* Available at: https://www.hsj.co.uk/bath-and-north-east-somerset-swindon-and-wiltshire-ics/private-provider-takes-over-nhs-services-worth-13bn/7037994.article (Accessed: 12 March 2025).

The King's Fund (2019) Is the NHS being privatised?, *The King's Fund.* Available at: https://www.kingsfund.org.uk/publications/articles/big-election-questions-nhs-privatised (Accessed: 14 August 2020).

Thomas, C. (2020) *Resilient Health and Care: Learning the Lessons of Covid-19 in the English NHS.* London: Institute for Public Policy Research.

Thomas, Chris (2022) 'The buy-out is the existential threat to the NHS', *Health Service Journal.* Available at: https://www.hsj.co.uk/policy-and-regulation/the-buy-out-is-the-existential-threat-to-the-nhs/7031750.article (Accessed: 7 March 2025).

Thomas, Christopher (2022) *The Five Health Frontiers: A New Radical Blueprint.* London: Pluto Press.

Thompson, E. P. (1965) 'The peculiarities of the English', *The Socialist Register*, 2: 311–362. Available at: https://socialistregister.com/index.php/srv/article/view/5963/2859.

Thompson, E. P. (1980) *The Making of the English Working Class.* London: Penguin Books.

Thompson, E. P. (1987) 'Diary: on the NHS', *London Review of Books*, 9(9).

Thompson, E. P. (1991a) 'The Moral Economy of the English Crowd in the Eighteenth Century', in E. P. Thompson (ed.) *Customs in Common.* London: Penguin Books, pp 185–258.

Thompson, E. P. (1991b) 'The Moral Economy Reviewed', in *Customs in Common.* London: Penguin Books, pp 259–351.

Tidman, Z. (2024) 'Revealed: the ongoing impact of delays to 'new hospital' schemes', *Health Service Journal.* Available at: https://www.hsj.co.uk/finance-and-efficiency/revealed-the-ongoing-impact-of-delays-to-new-hospital-schemes/7038060.article (Accessed: 6 March 2025).

Timmins, N. (2018) *'The World's Biggest Quango': The First Five Years of NHS England.* London: The King's Fund.

Timmins, N. and Baird, B. (2022) *The Covid-19 vaccination programme: trials, tribulations and successes*, The King's Fund. Available at: https://www.kingsfund.org.uk/insight-and-analysis/reports/covid-19-vaccination-programme (Accessed: 5 March 2025).

Todd, S. (2014) *The People: The Rise and Fall of the Working Class.* London: John Murray.

Toffolutti, V., Reeves, A., McKee, M. and Stuckler, D. (2017) 'Outsourcing cleaning services increases MRSA incidence: evidence from 126 english acute trusts', *Social Science and Medicine*, 174: 64–69. doi: 10.1016/j.socscimed.2016.12.015.

Tomkow, L. (2019) *Health and Ageing in a Hostile Environment: Understanding Older Asylum Applicants' Narratives of Life, Health and Ageing in the UK*. Manchester: University of Manchester.

Tomkow, L. J. et al. (2020) 'Healthcare access for asylum seekers and refugees in England: a mixed methods study exploring service users' and health care professionals' awareness', *European Journal of Public Health*, 30(3): 527–532. doi: 10.1093/eurpub/ckz193.

Travis, A. (2013) Theresa May defends plans to create 'hostile environment', *The Guardian*. Available at: https://www.theguardian.com/politics/2013/oct/10/immigration-bill-theresa-may-hostile-environment (Accessed: 24 August 2020).

Trnka, S. and Trundle, C. (2017) 'Introduction. Competing Responsibilities: Reckoning Personal Responsibility, Care for the Other, and the Social Contract in Contemporary Life', in Trnka, S. and Trundle, C. (eds) *Competing Responsibilities: The Politics and Ethics of Contemporary Life*. Durham, NC: Duke University Press, pp 1–24. doi: 10.1215/9780822373056.

Wainwright, H. (2015) *My support for Jeremy Corbyn is about much more than 'reclaiming Labour'*, *Red Pepper*. Available at: http://www.redpepper.org.uk/my-support-for-jeremy-corbyn-is-about-much-more-than-reclaiming-labour/ (Accessed: 31 July 2019).

Walker, D. and Tizard, J. (2018) *Out of Contract: Time to Move on From the 'Love In' with Outsourcing and PFI*. London: The Smith Institute.

Walsh, D., Dundas, R., McCartney, G., Gibson, M. and Seaman, R. (2022) 'Bearing the burden of austerity: how do changing mortality rates in the UK compare between men and women?', *Journal of Epidemiology and Community Health*, 76(12): 1027–1033. doi: 10.1136/jech-2022-219645.

Walshe, K., Lorne, C., Coleman, A., McDonald, R. and Turner, A. (2018) *Devolving Health and Social Care: Learning from Greater Manchester*. Manchester: The University of Manchester.

Watkins, J., Wulaningsih, W., Da Zhou, C., Marshall, D., Sylianteng, G., Dela Rosa, P., et al. (2017) 'Effects of health and social care spending constraints on mortality in England: a time trend analysis', *BMJ Open*, 7(11). doi: 10.1136/bmjopen-2017-017722.

Watkins, S. (1987) *Medicine and Labour – The Politics of a Profession*. London: Lawrence and Wishart.

Webster, C. (2002) *The National Health Service: A Political History*. Oxford: Oxford University Press.

Whittle, H. J., Kiely, E., Millard, I., Jadhav, S. and Killaspy, H. (2024) 'The relational institution: an ethnographic study of recovery orientation and relational engagement on a psychiatric rehabilitation ward in London', *BMC Psychiatry*, 24(1): 738. doi: 10.1186/s12888-024-06140-0.

Wickens, C. (2022) *Provider collaboratives: explaining their role in system working*, The King's Fund. Available at: https://www.kingsfund.org.uk/insight-and-analysis/long-reads/provider-collaboratives (Accessed: 12 March 2025).

Wills, V. (2024) *Marx's Ethical Vision*. Oxford: Oxford University Press.

Wilson, D. (2012) 'Who guards the guardians? Ian Kennedy, bioethics and the "ideology of accountability" in British medicine', *Social History of Medicine*, 25(1): 193–211. doi: 10.1093/shm/hkr090.

Wilson, D. (2015) *The Making of British Bioethics*. Manchester: Manchester University Press. doi: 10.7228/manchester/9781847798879.

Winant, G. (2019) *Professional-Managerial Chasm: A Sociological Designation Turned into an Epithet and Hurled like a Missile, n+1*. Available at: https://nplusonemag.com/online-only/online-only/professional-managerial-chasm/ (Accessed: 18 June 2020).

Winant, G. (2021) *The Next Shift: The Fall of Industry and the Rise of Health Care in Rust Belt America*. Cambridge: Harvard University Press.

Wise, J. (2021) 'Covid-19: Ten Conservative MPs and peers referred companies to "VIP lane" that won £1.6bn of PPE contracts', *BMJ*, 375(November): n2825. doi: 10.1136/bmj.n2825.

Wolfson, S. (2025) *National Health Service or National Safe Haven*. London: Policy Exchange.

Worthing, K. et al. (2023) 'Reluctance of general practice staff to register patients without documentation: a qualitative study in North East London', *British Journal of General Practice*, 73(729): E276–E283. doi: 10.3399/BJGP.2022.0336.

Wright, E. O. (2013) 'Transforming Capitalism through Real Utopias', *American Sociological Review*, 78(1): 1–25. doi: 10.1177/0003122412468882.

Yang, J. (2024) *Number of registered doctors in the United Kingdom (UK) in 2024, by gender and specialty, Statista*. Available at: https://www.statista.com/statistics/891945/general-practitioners-in-england-by-gender/ (Accessed: 12 March 2025).

Younis, T. and Jadhav, S. (2019) 'Keeping Our Mouths Shut: The Fear and Racialized Self-Censorship of British Healthcare Professionals in PREVENT Training', *Culture, Medicine, and Psychiatry*, 43(3): 404–424. doi: 10.1007/s11013-019-09629-6.

Younis, T. and Jadhav, S. (2020) 'Islamophobia in the National Health Service: an ethnography of institutional racism in PREVENT's counter-radicalisation policy', *Sociology of Health & Illness*, 42(3): 610–626. doi: 10.1111/1467-9566.13047.

Zelizer, V. A. (2005) *The Purchase of Intimacy*. Princeton, NJ: Princeton University Press.

Zhou, X., Correa, A., Palmer, T., Sun, M., Pizzo, E., Gomes, P. and Skordis, J. (2026) 'Earned settlement: the value of international health and care workers in the UK', *The Lancet Regional Health – Europe*, 62: 101596. doi: 10.1016/j.lanepe.2026.101596.

Index

References to endnotes show both the page number and the note number (170n7).

O

P